This Book Belongs To:

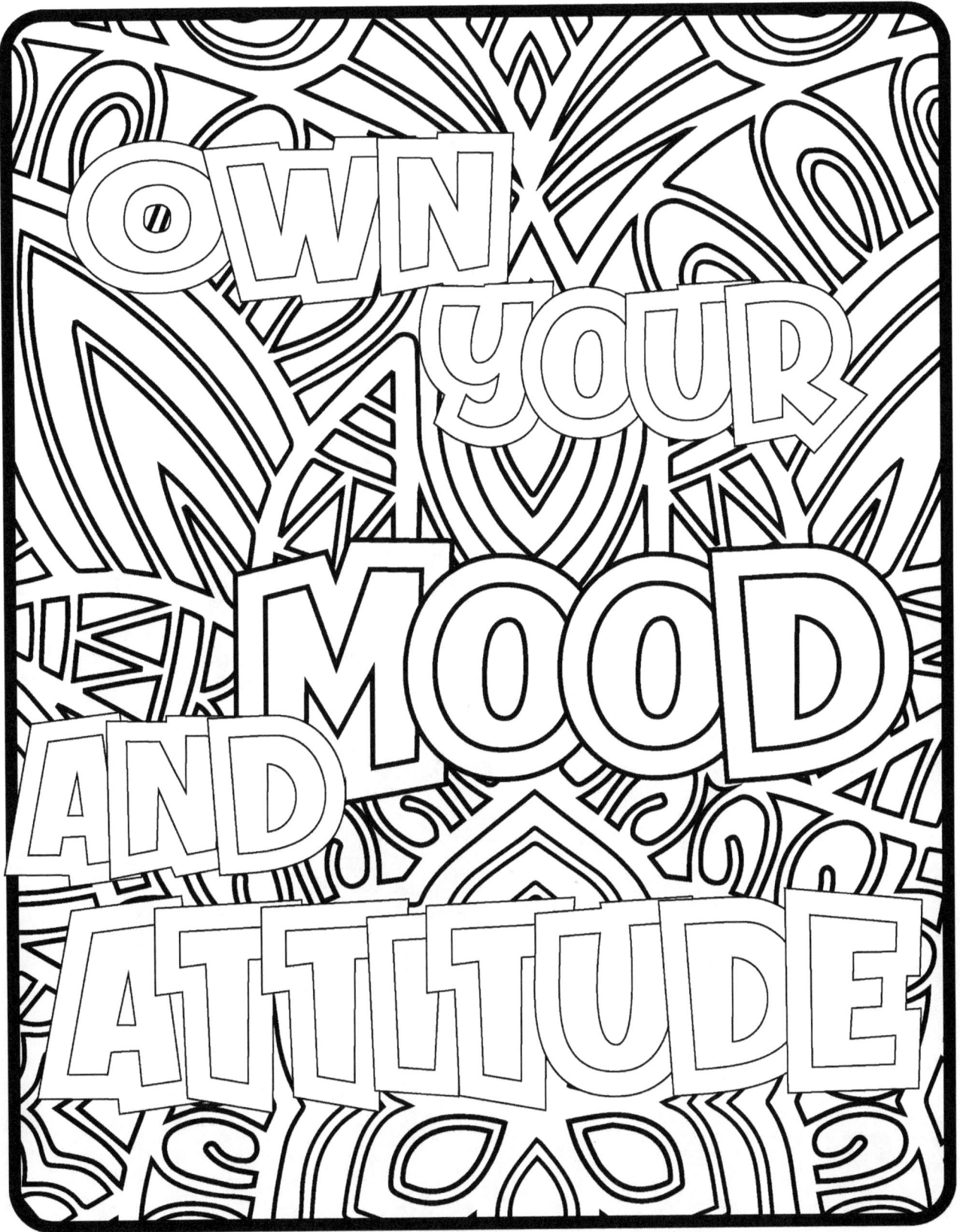

OWN YOUR MOOD AND ATTITUDE

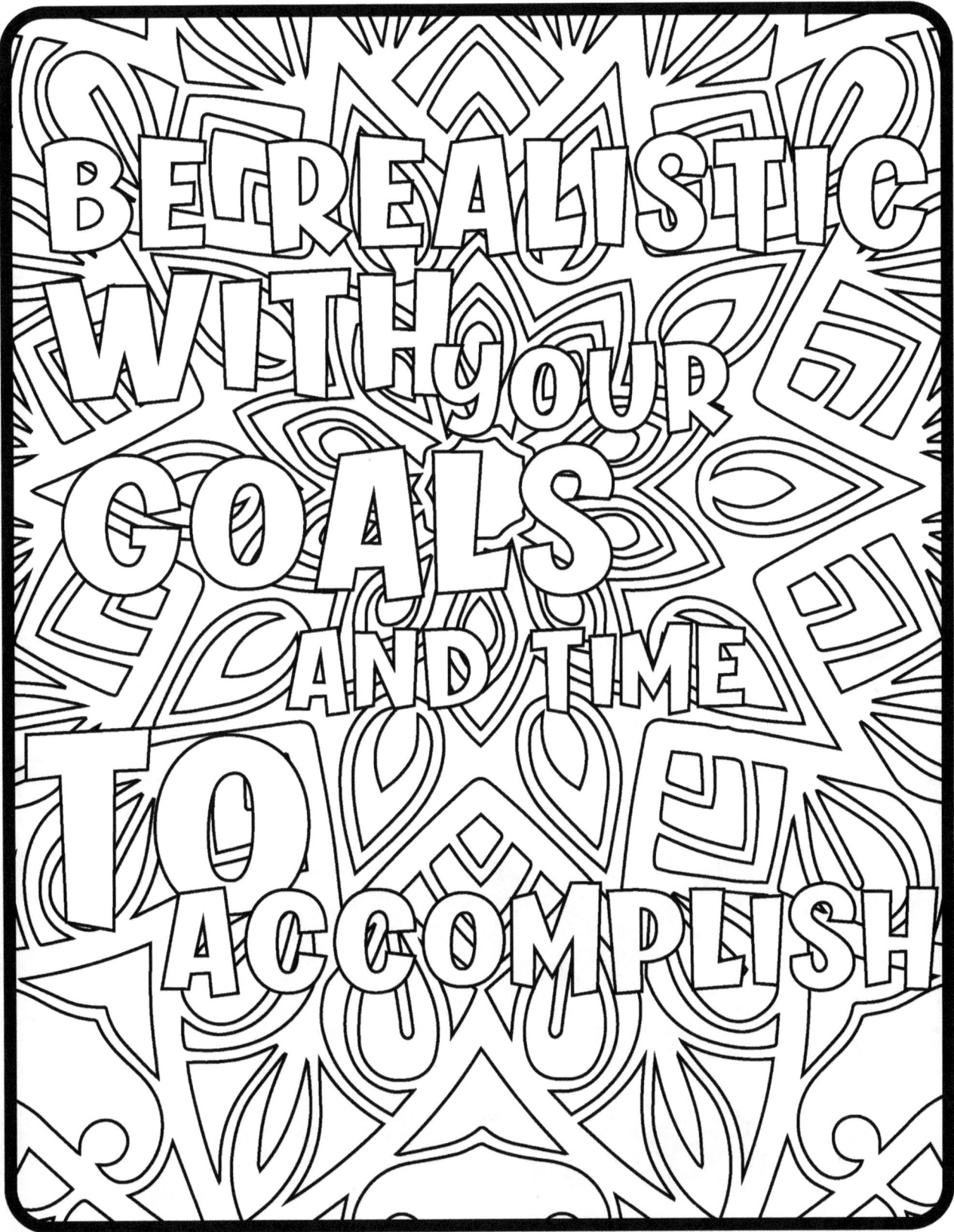

BE REALISTIC WITH YOUR GOALS AND TIME TO ACCOMPLISH

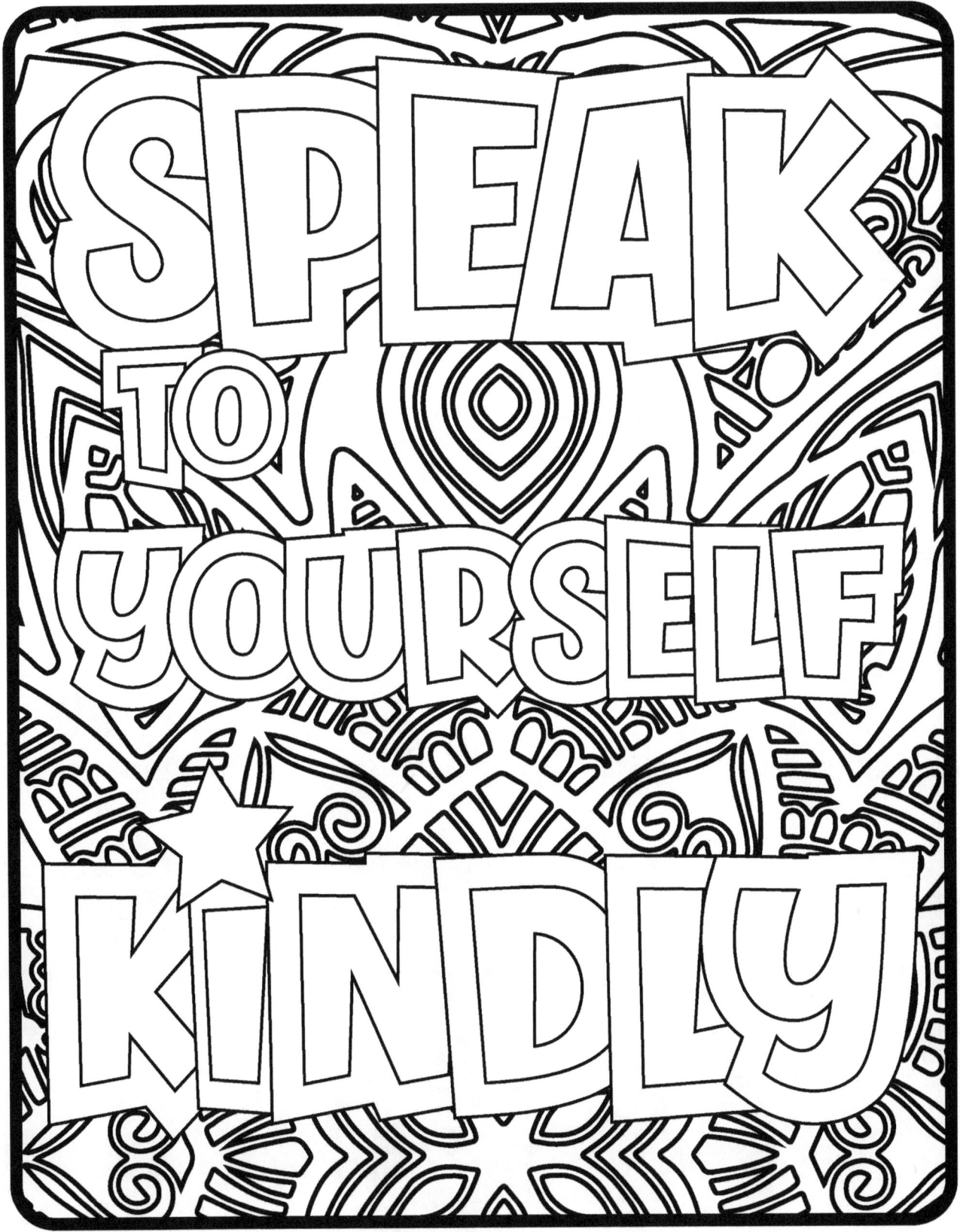

SPEAK TO YOURSELF KINDLY

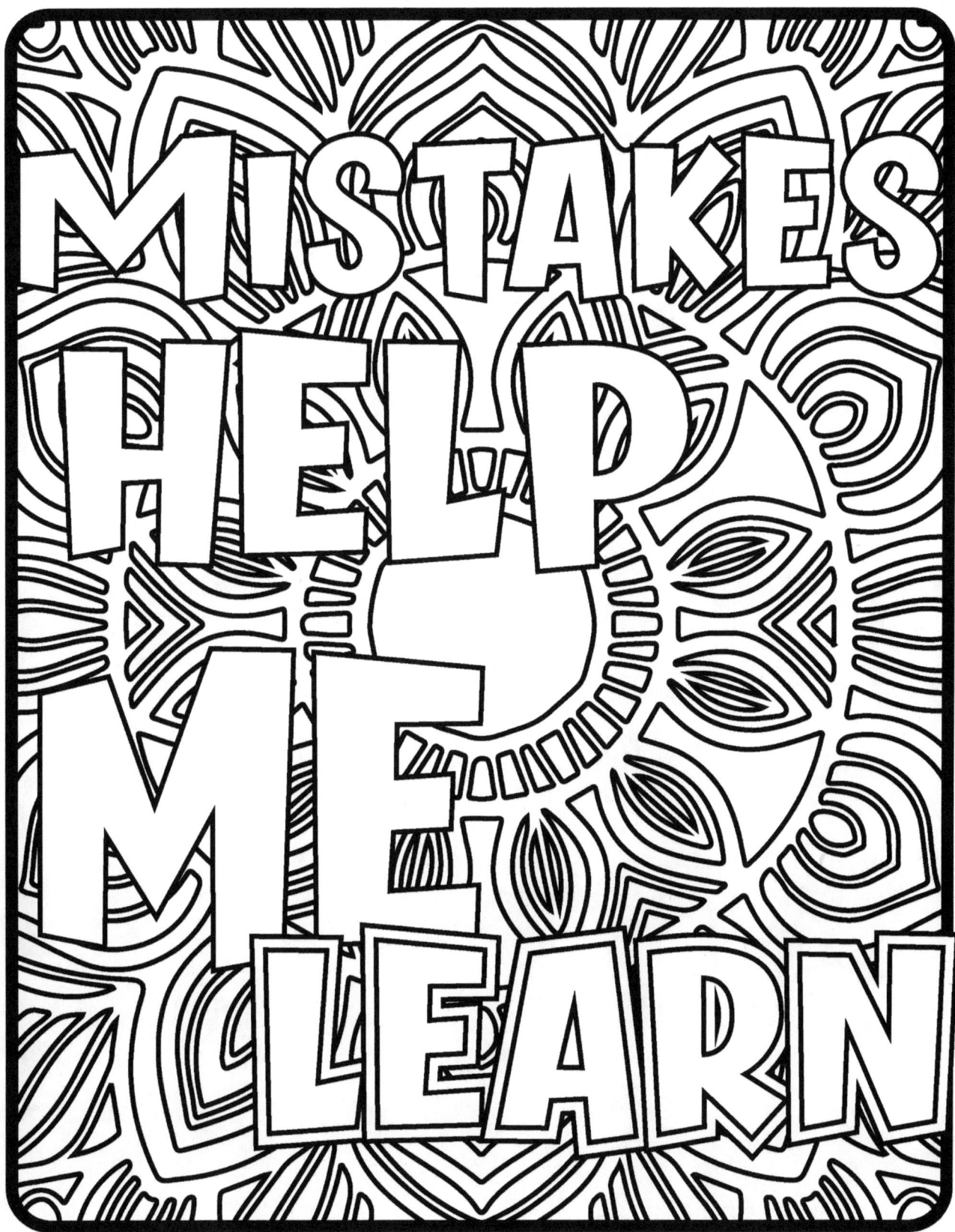

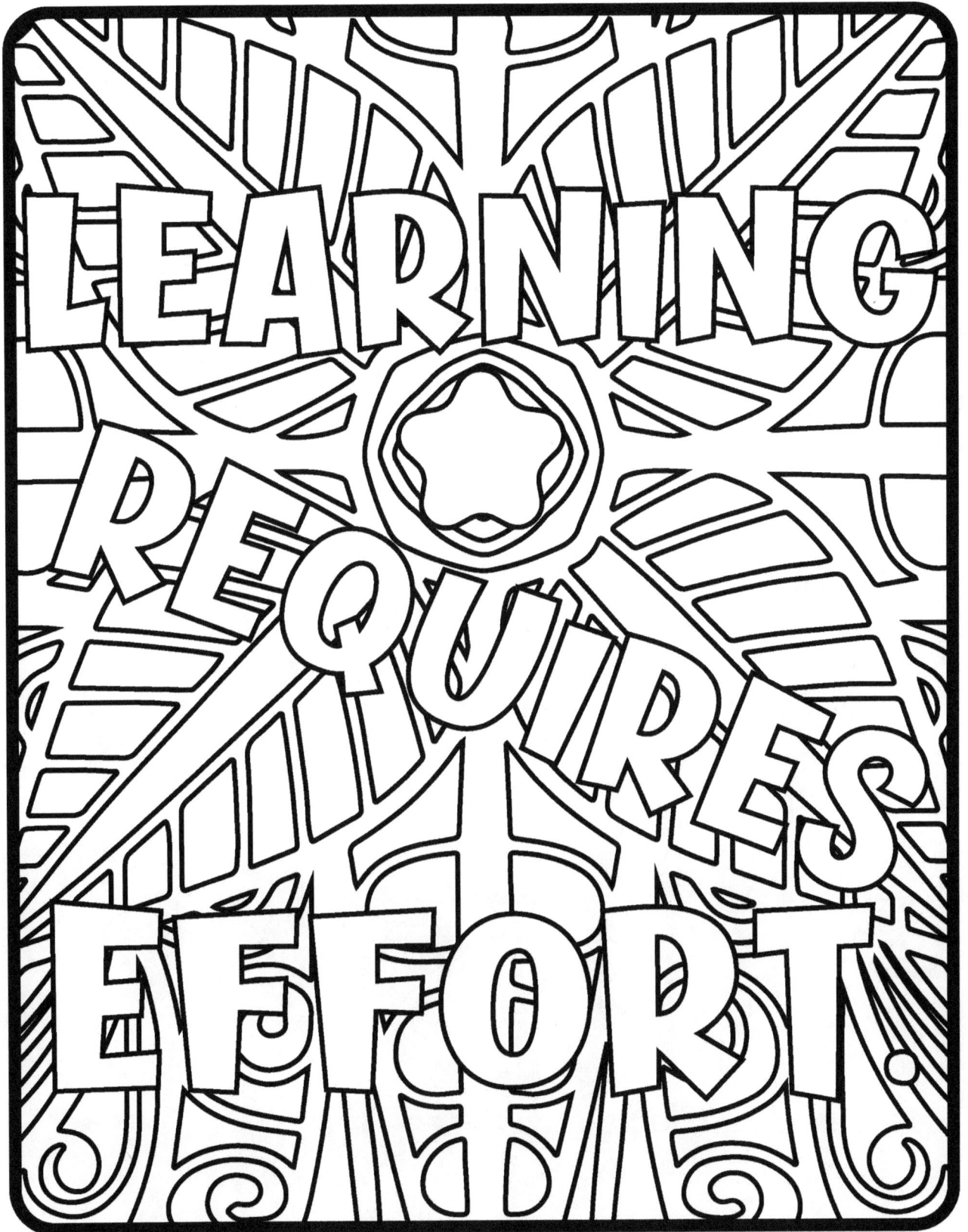

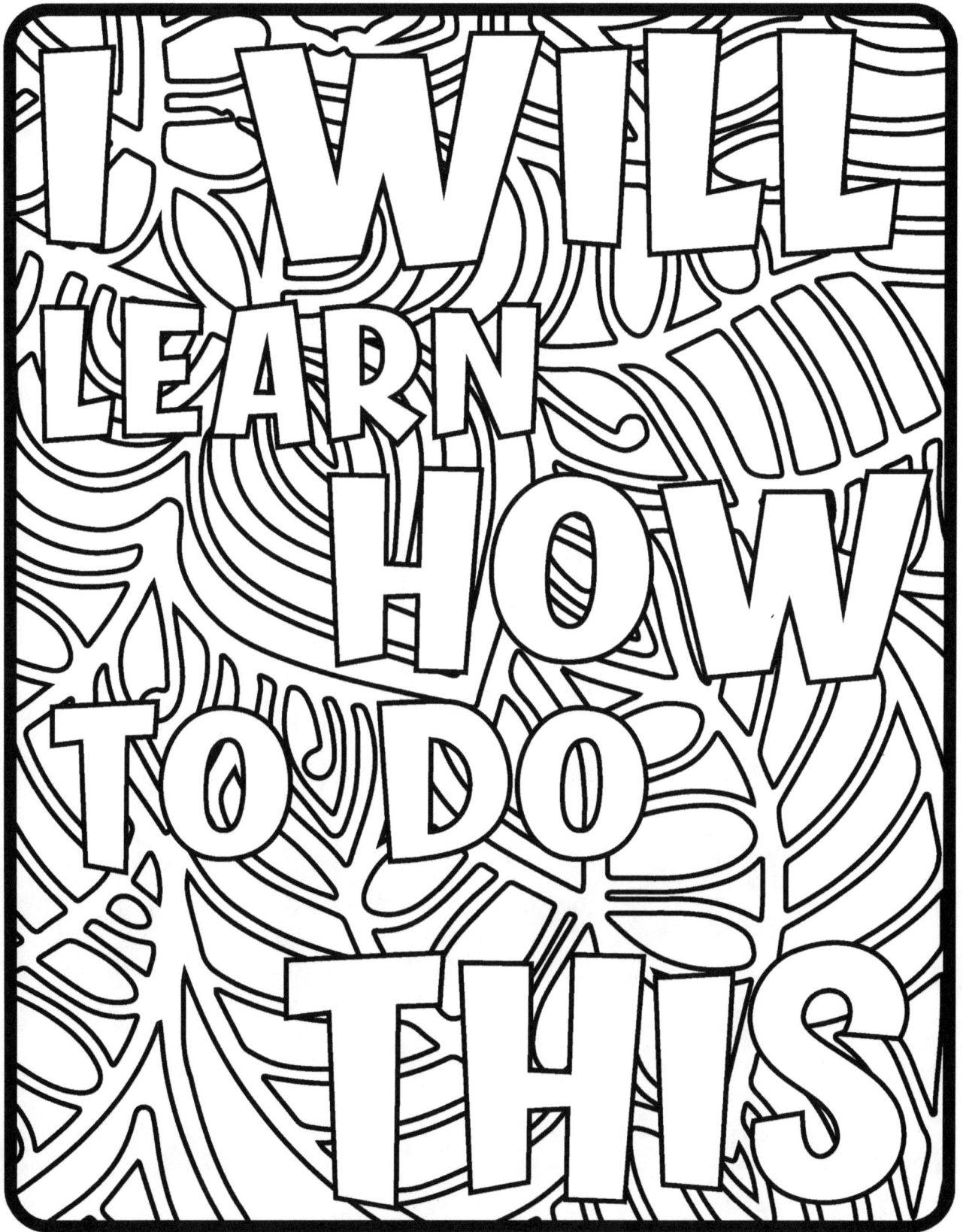

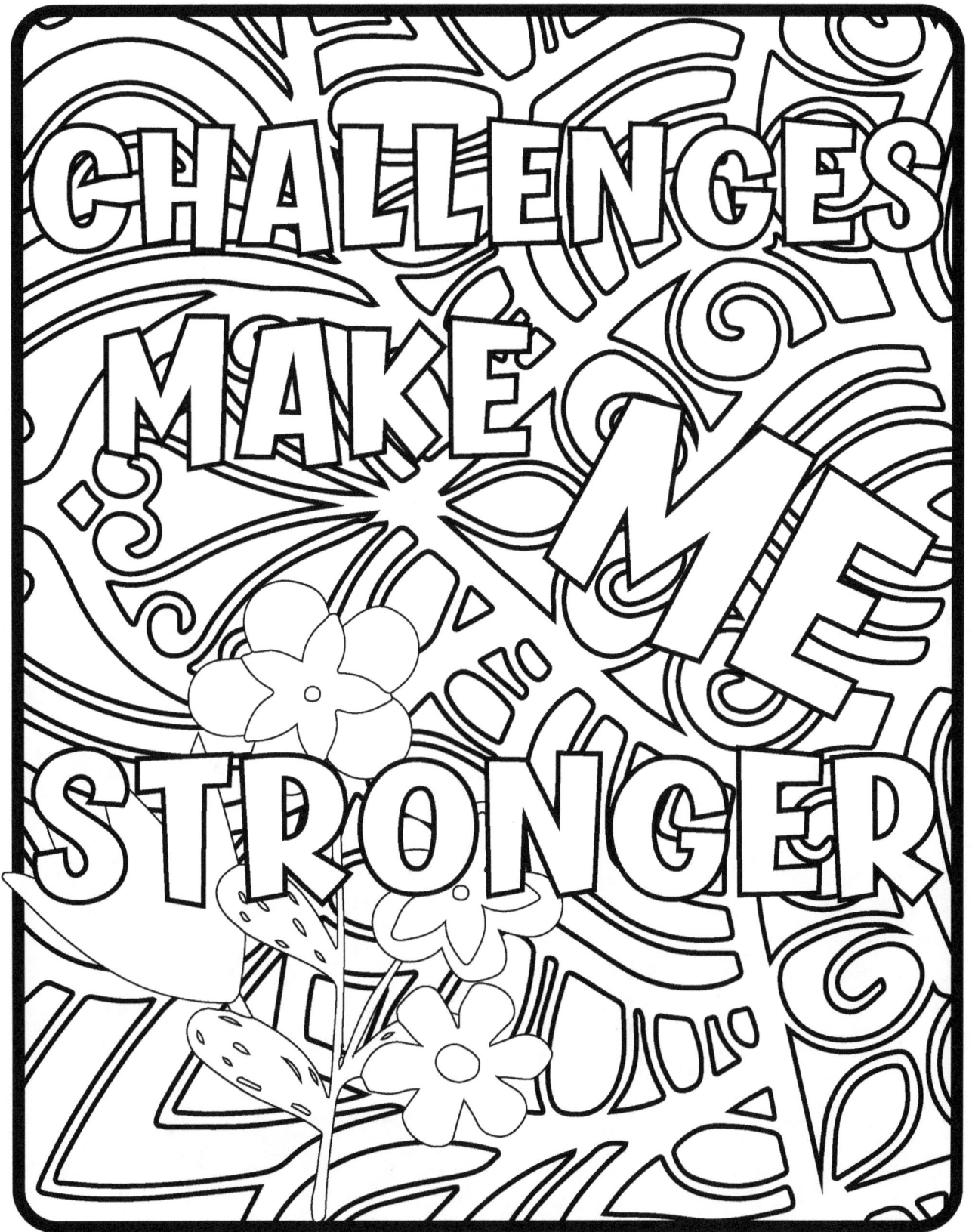

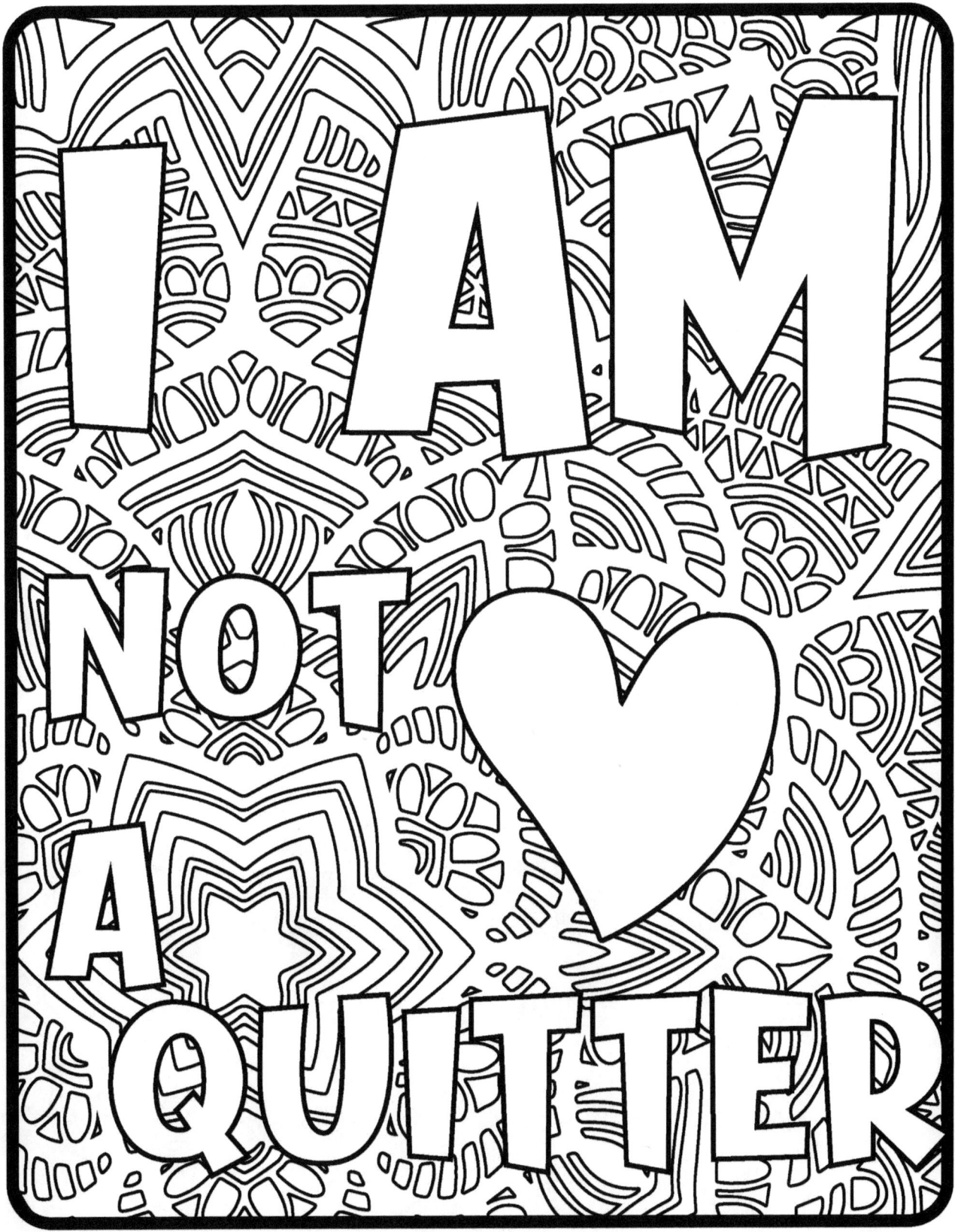

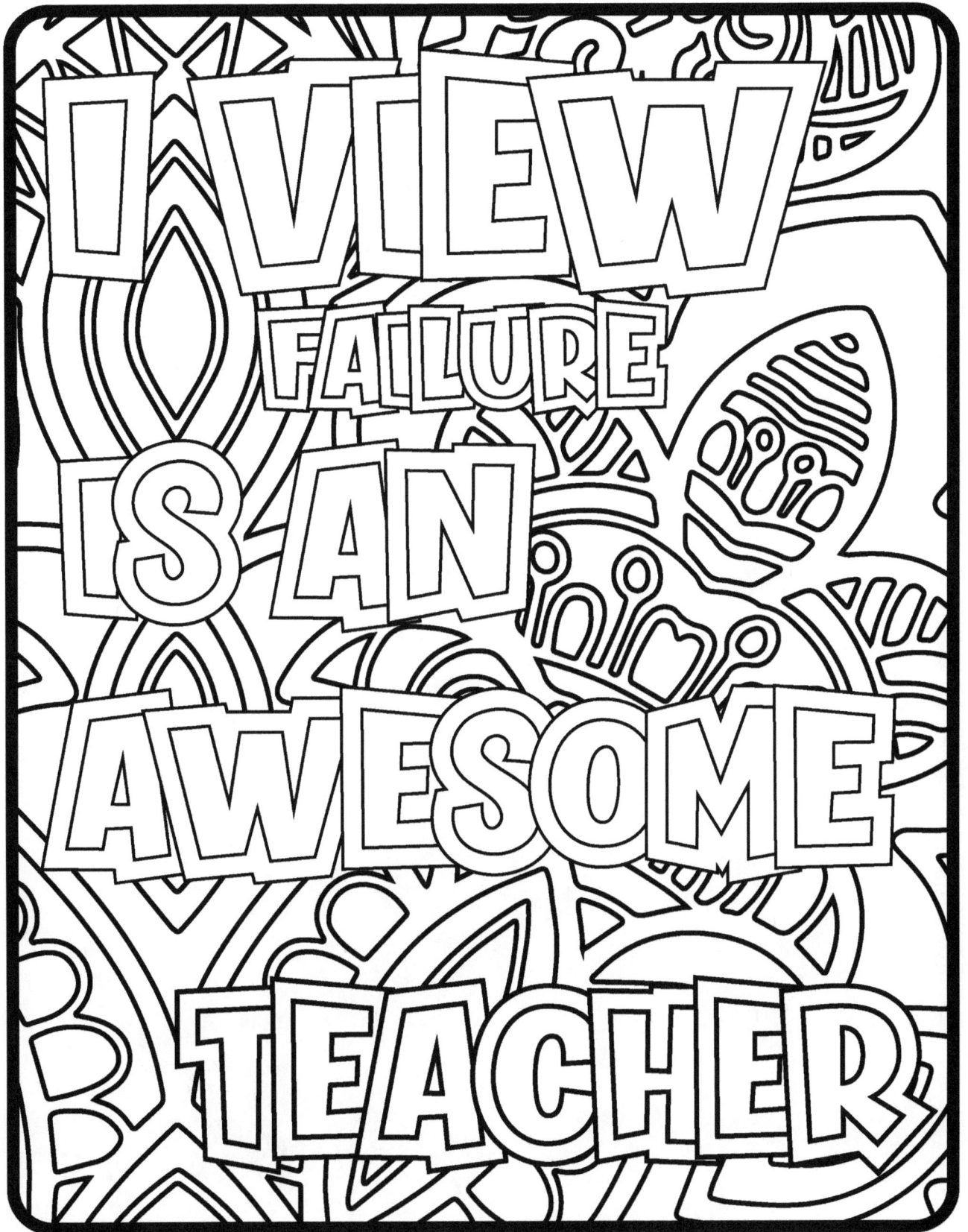

I VIEW FAILURE IS AN AWESOME TEACHER

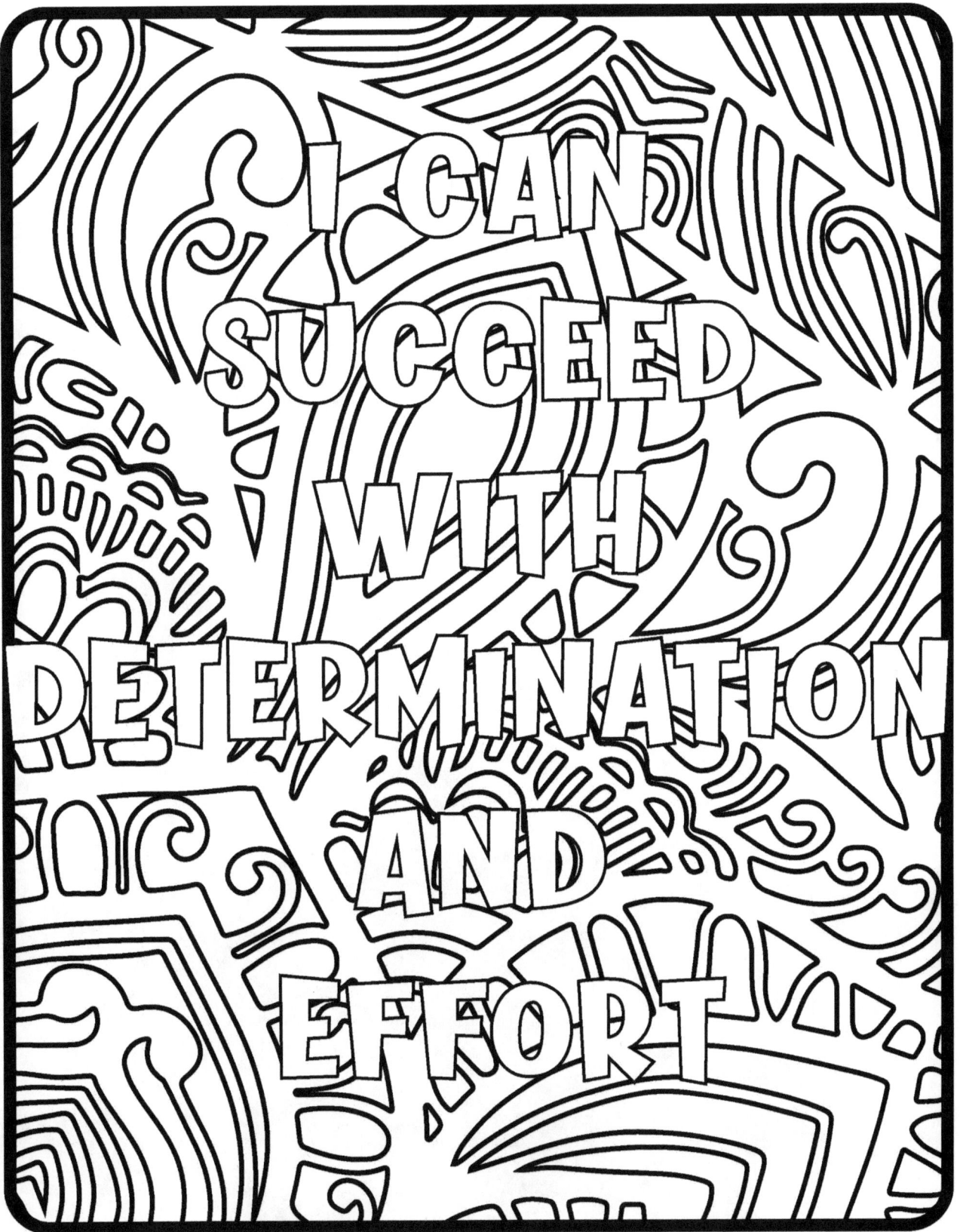

I CAN SUCCEED WITH DETERMINATION AND EFFORT

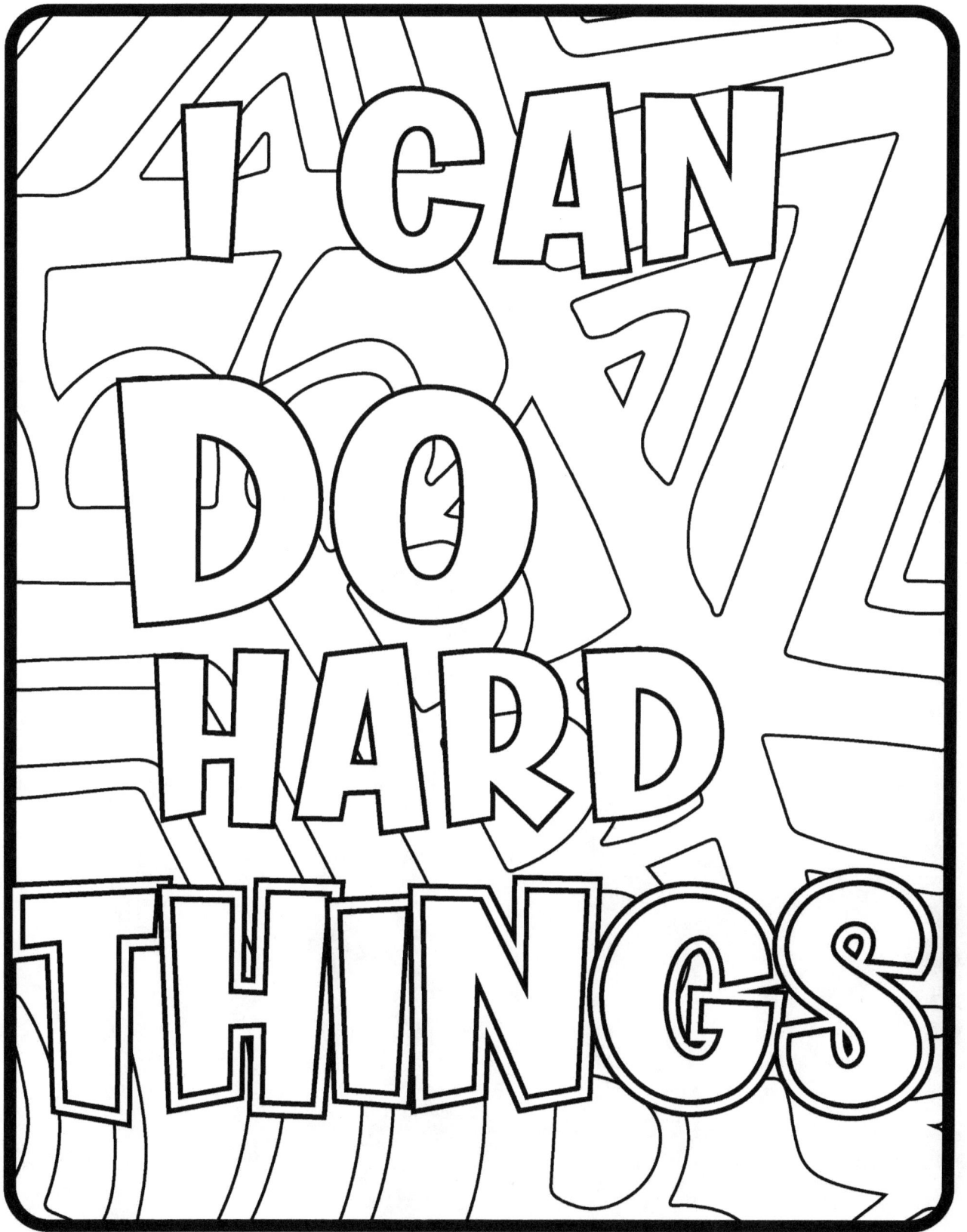

I CAN DO HARD THINGS

CRITICISM HELPS ME BECOME BETTER

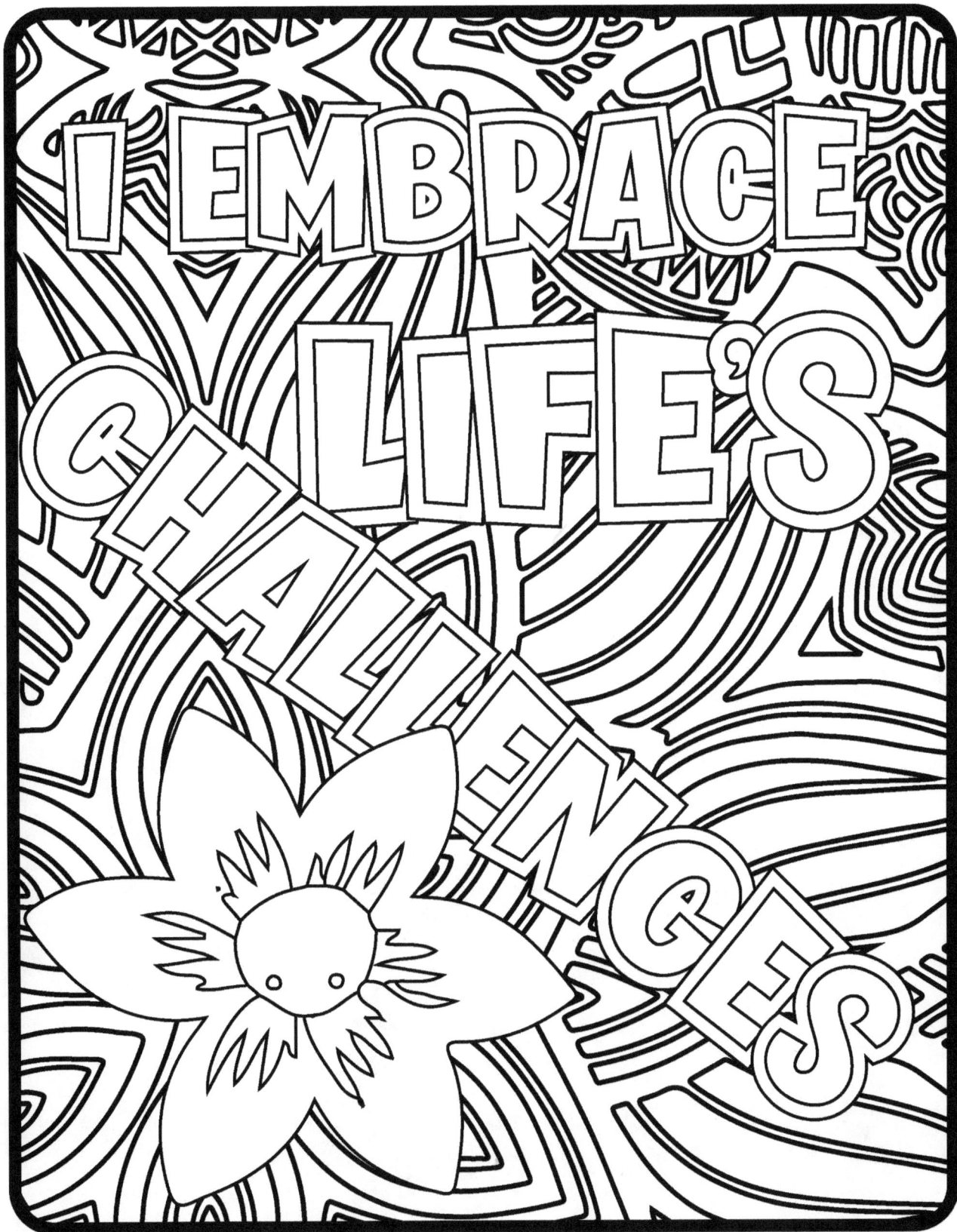

I EMBRACE LIFE'S CHALLENGES

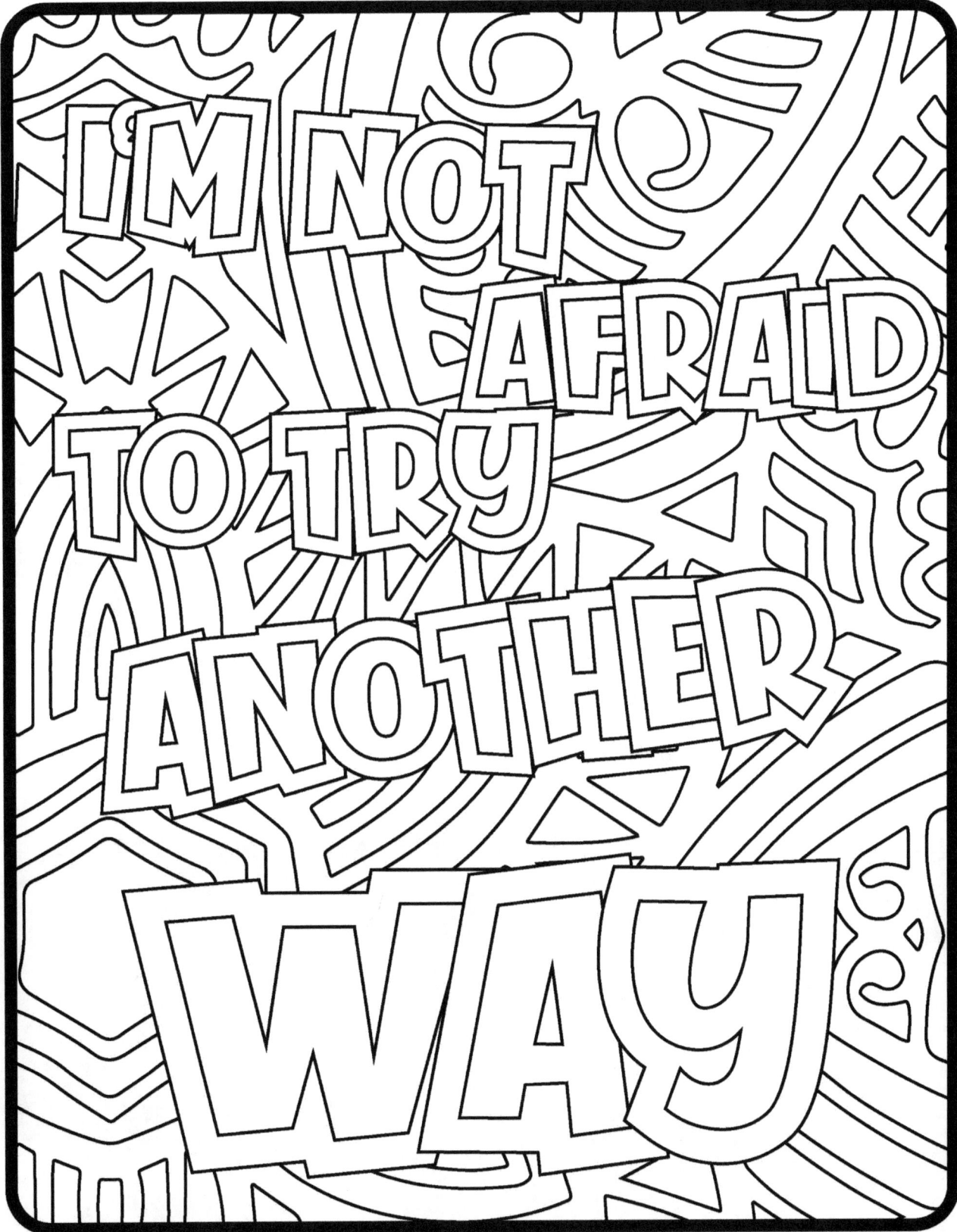

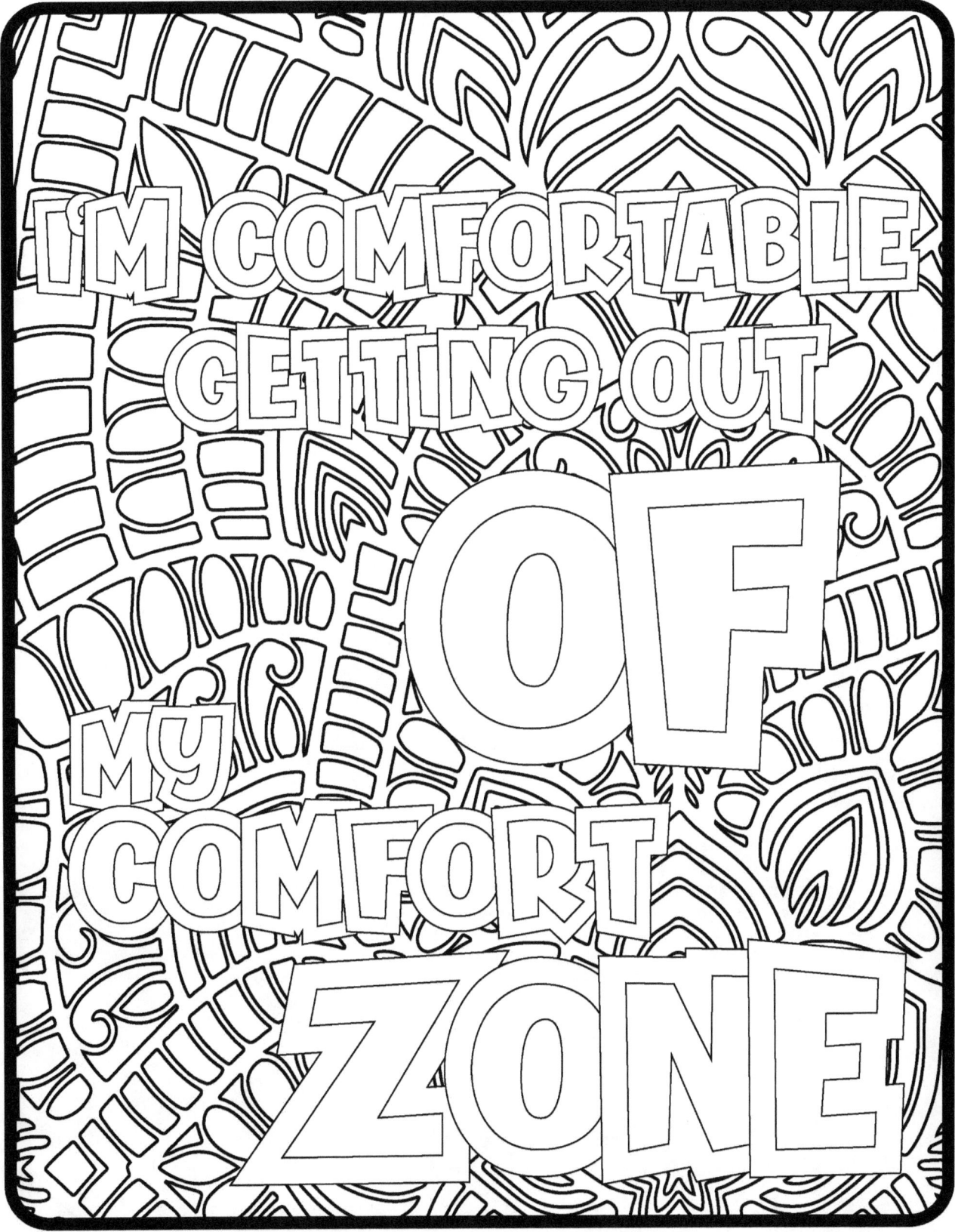

I'M COMFORTABLE GETTING OUT OF MY COMFORT ZONE

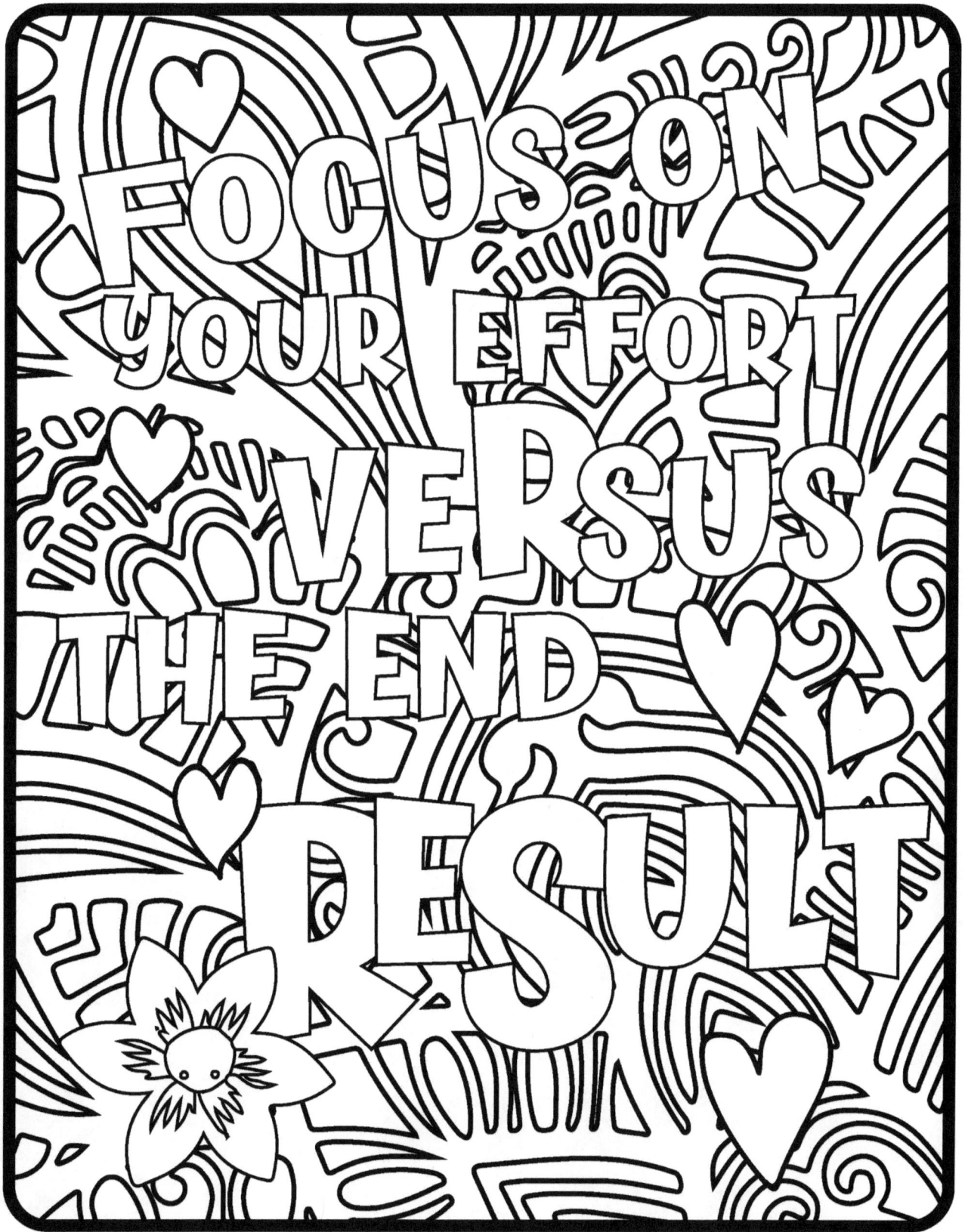

FOCUS ON YOUR EFFORT VERSUS THE END RESULT

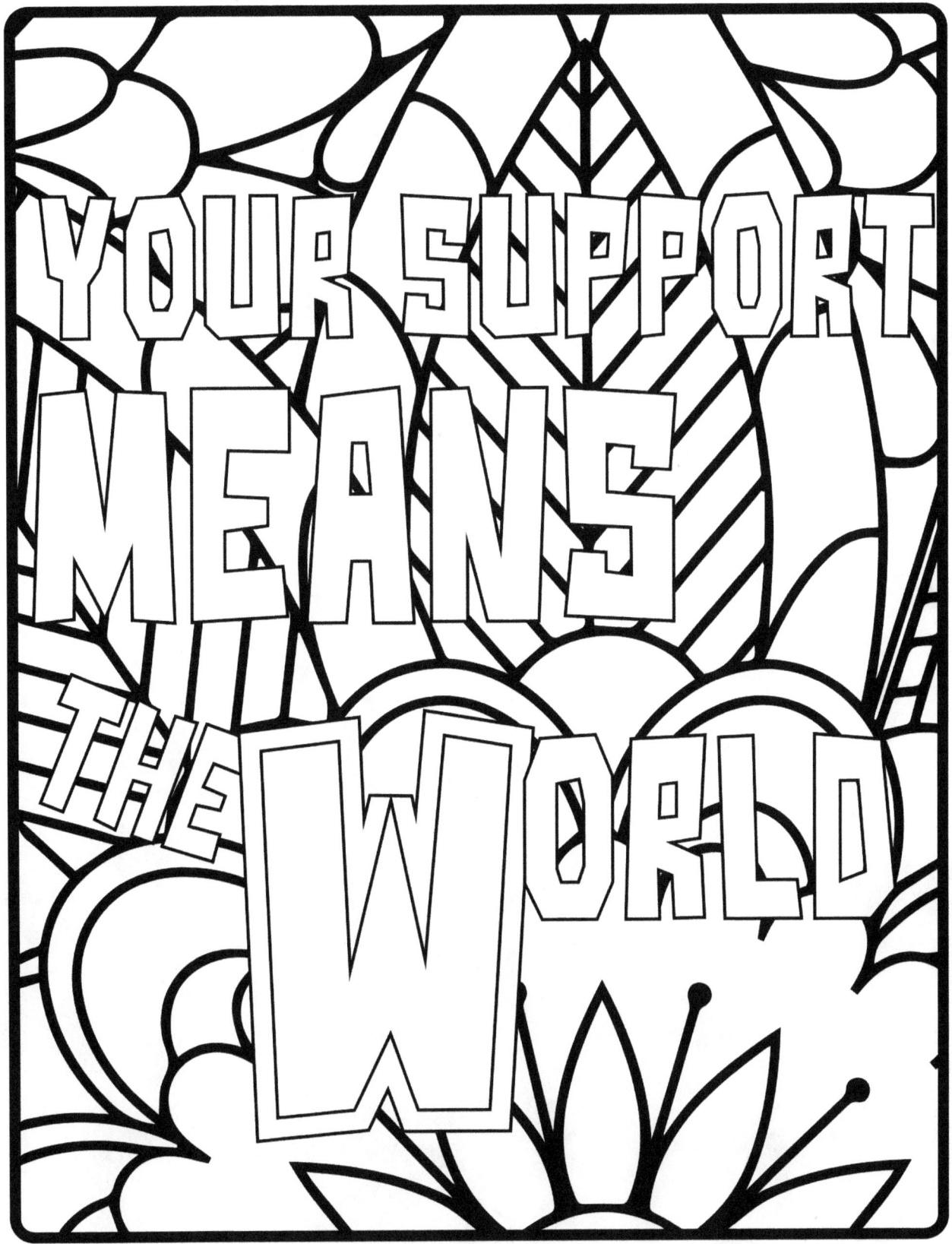

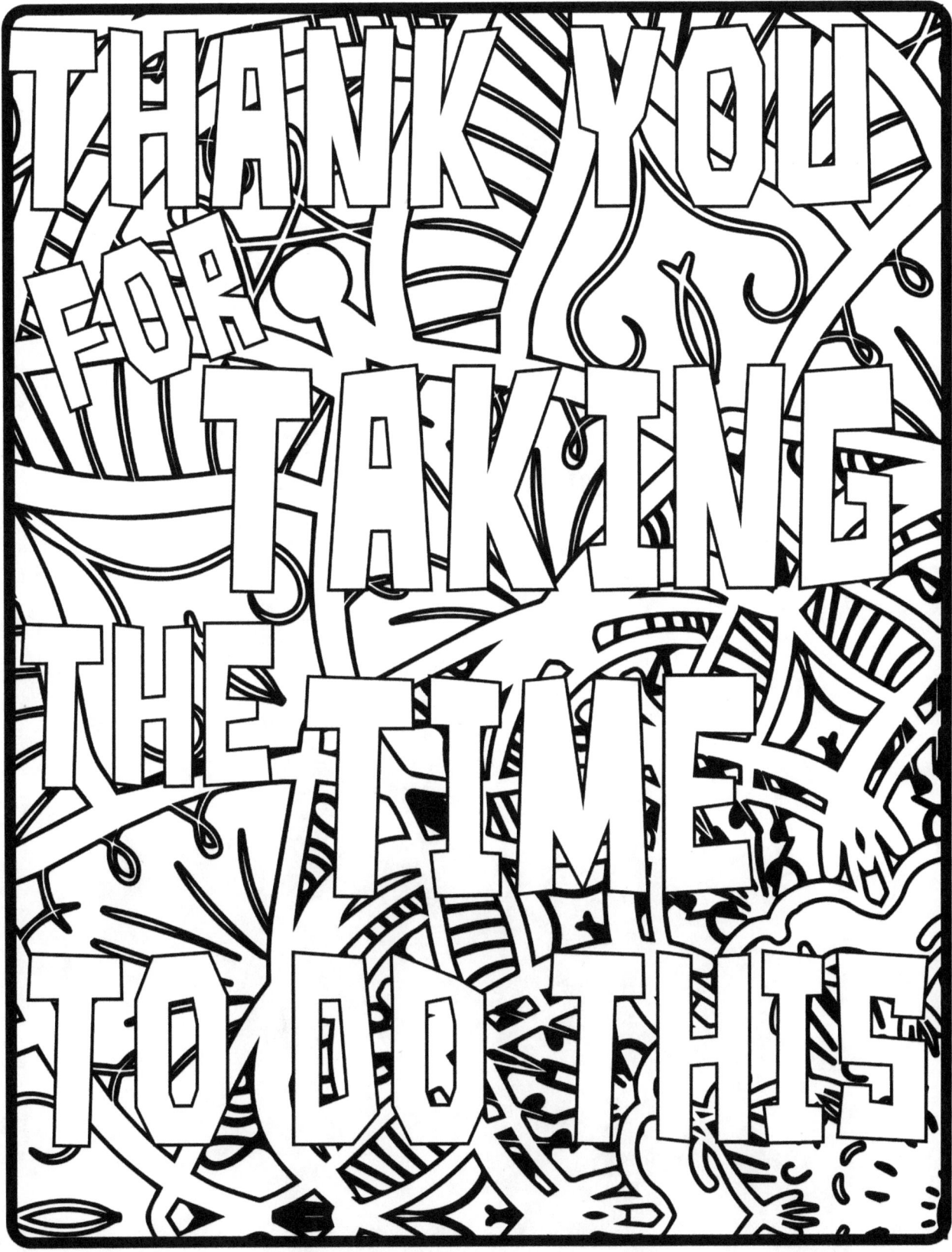

THANK YOU FOR TAKING THE TIME TO DO THIS

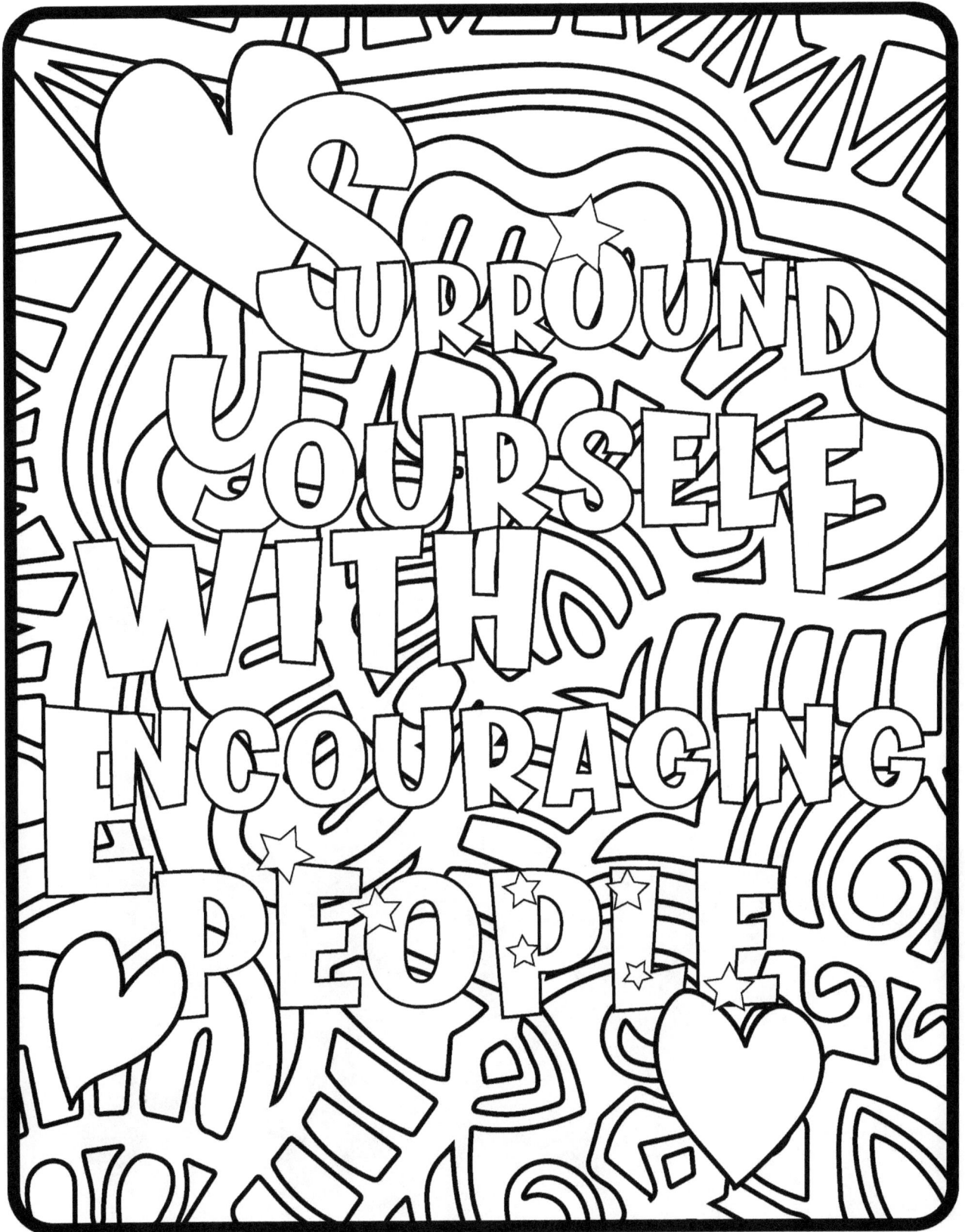
SURROUND YOURSELF WITH ENCOURAGING PEOPLE

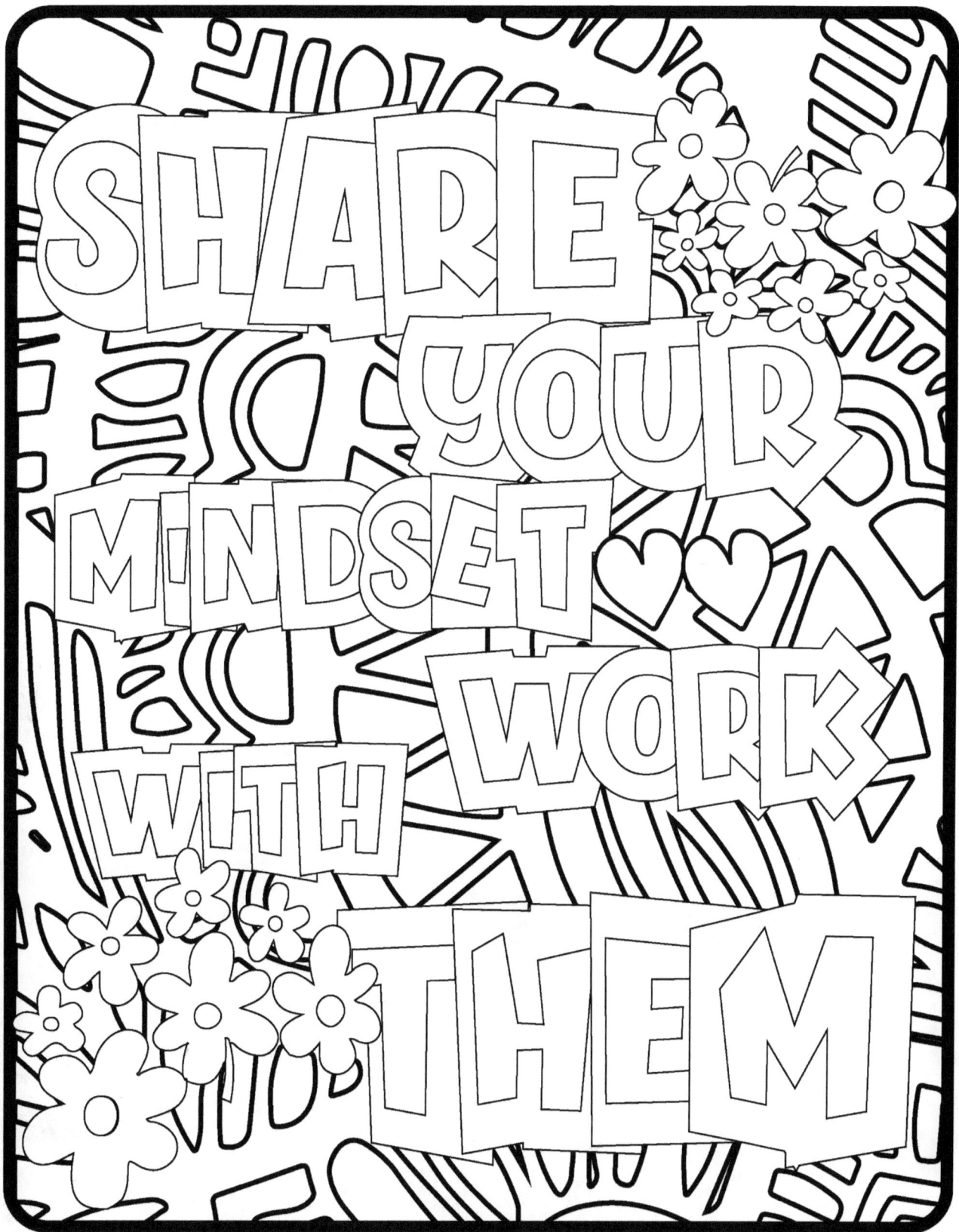

SHARE YOUR MINDSET WORK WITH THEM

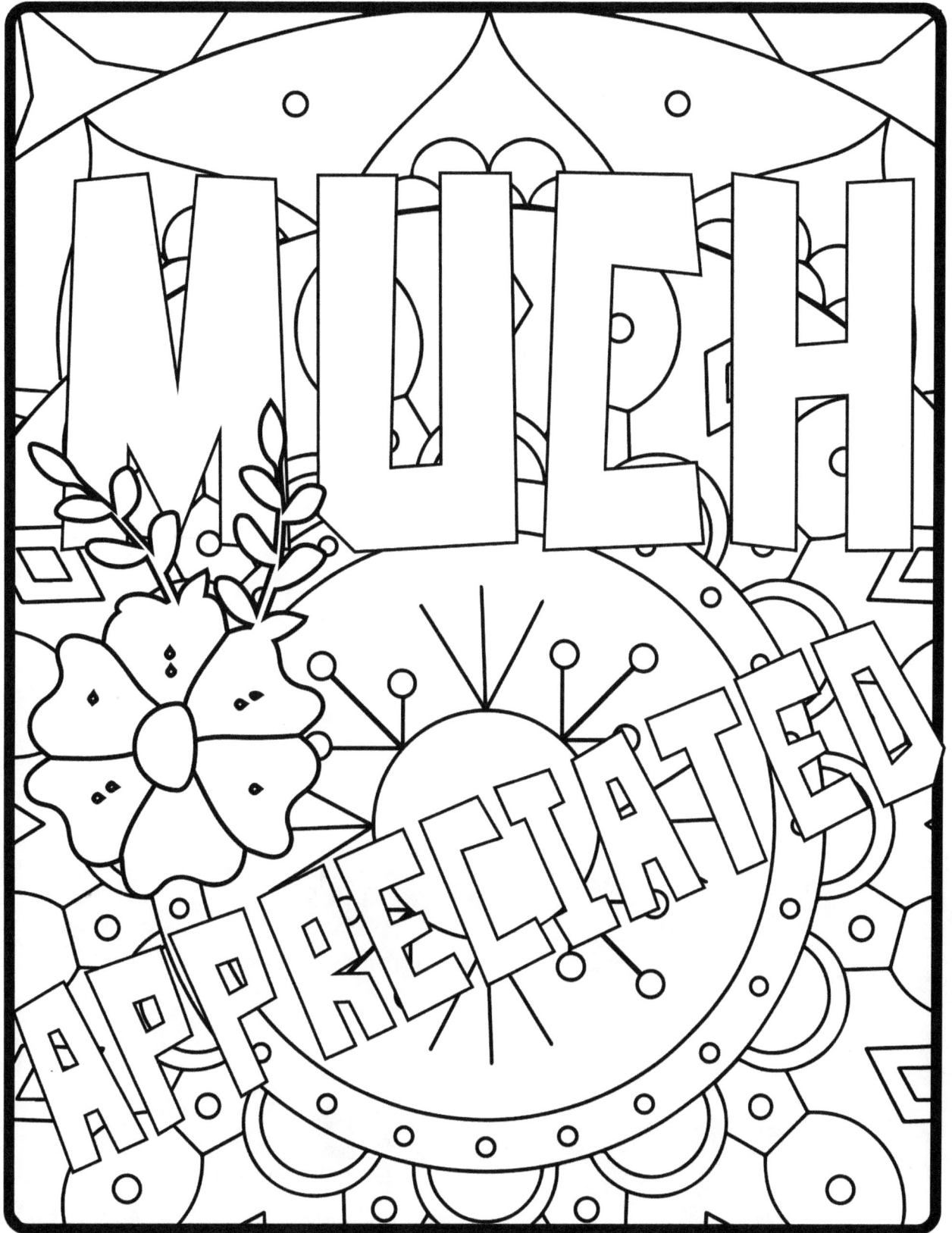

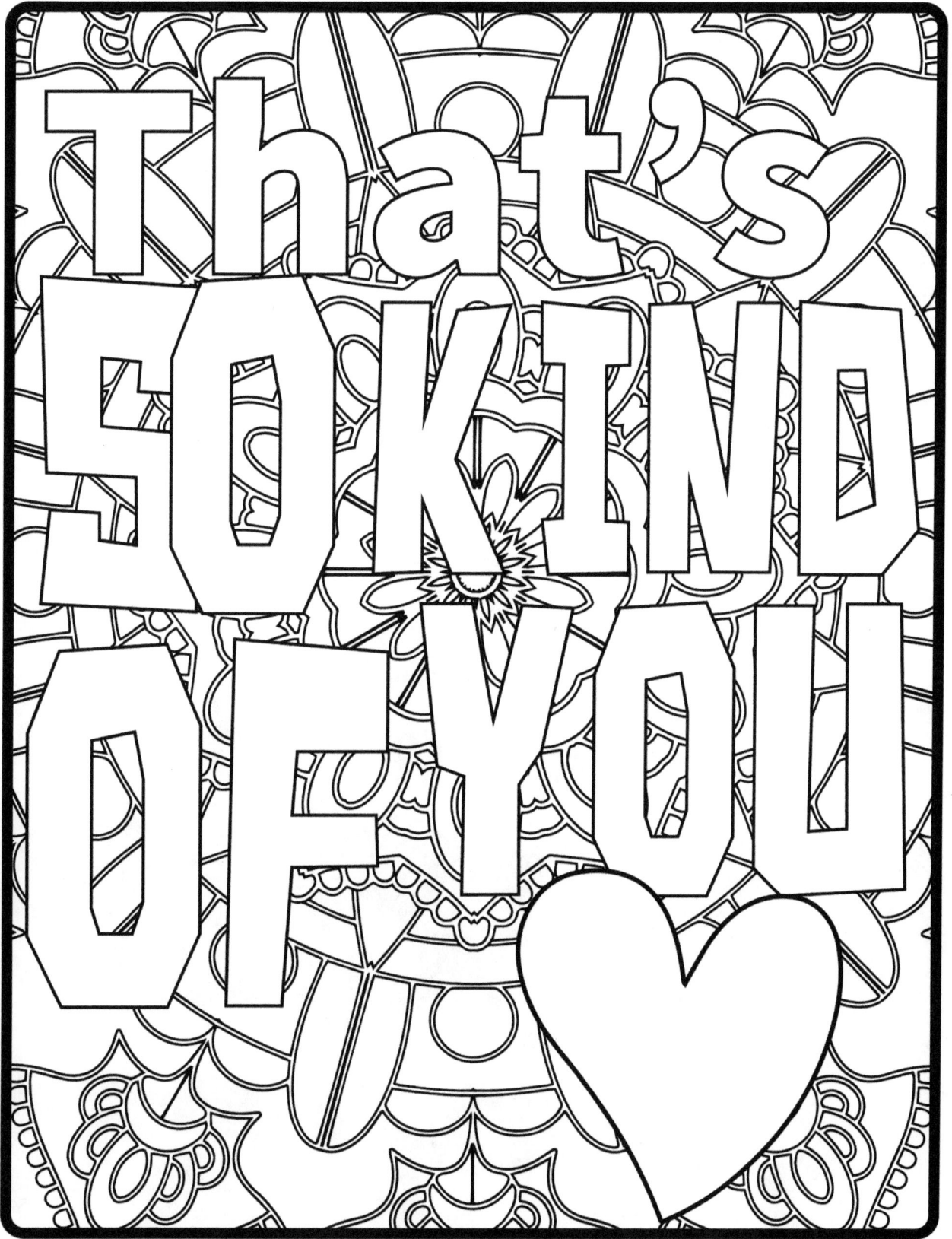

That's SO KIND OF YOU

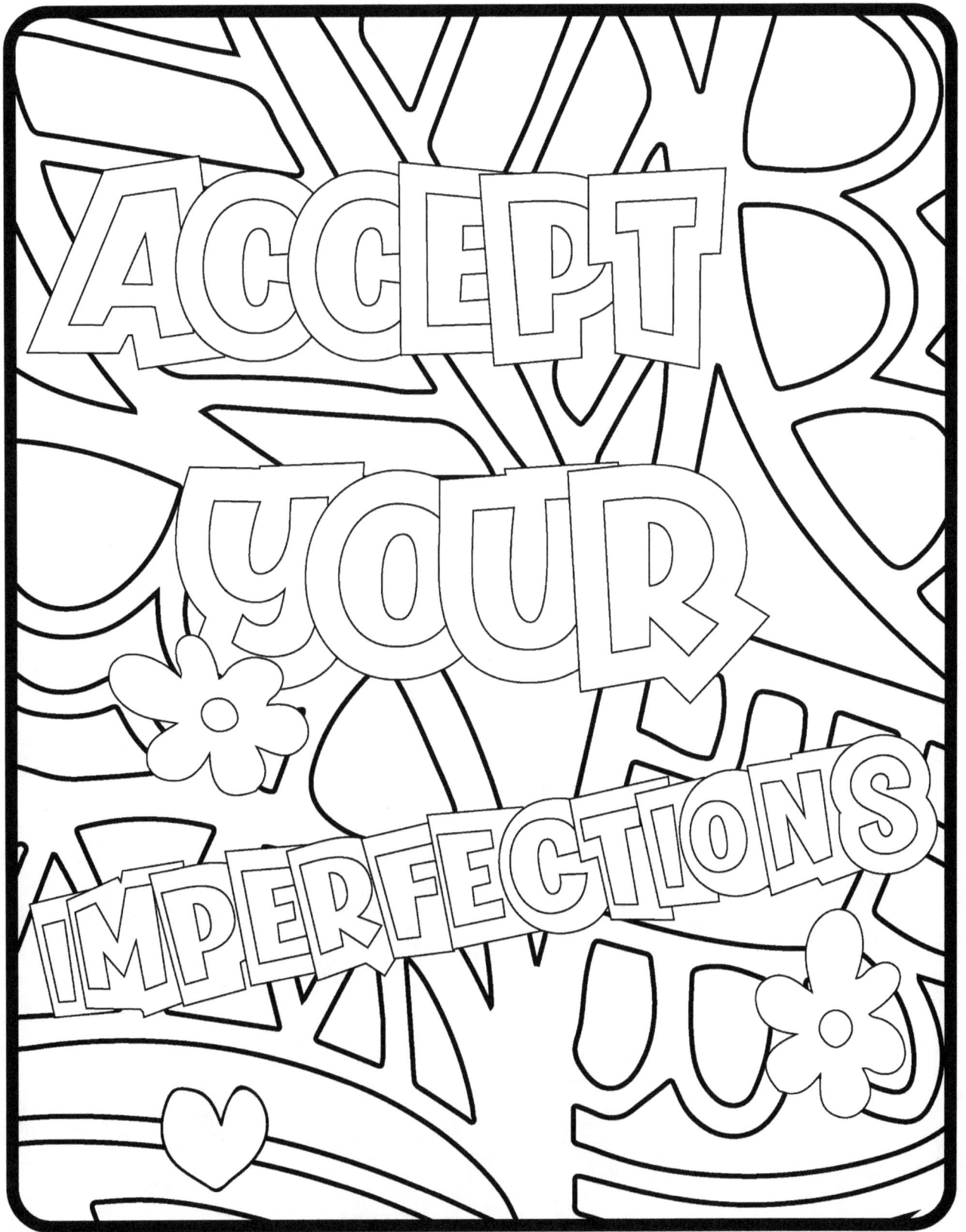

BELIEVE CHANGE AND IMPROVEMENT ARE POSSIBLE

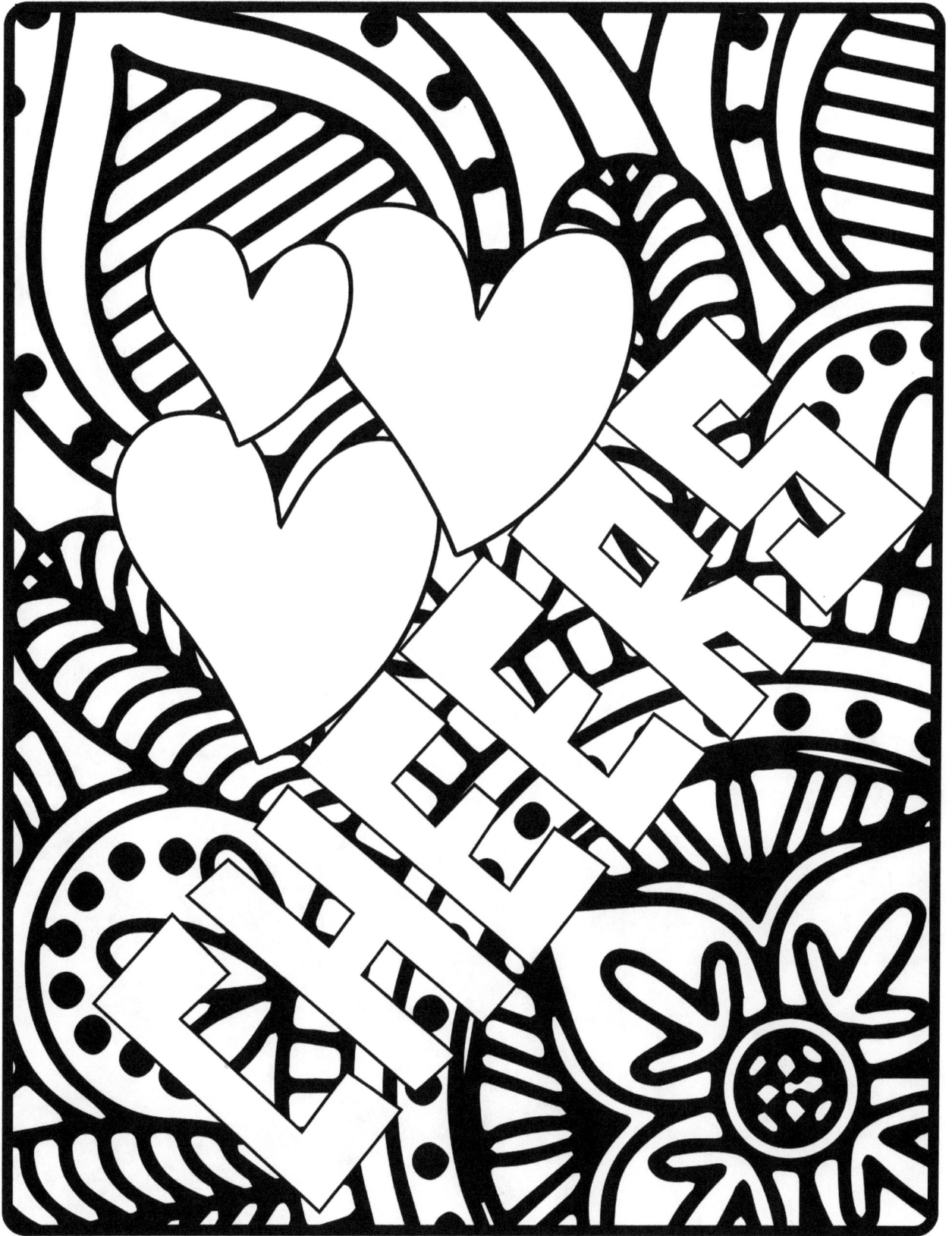

CHEERS

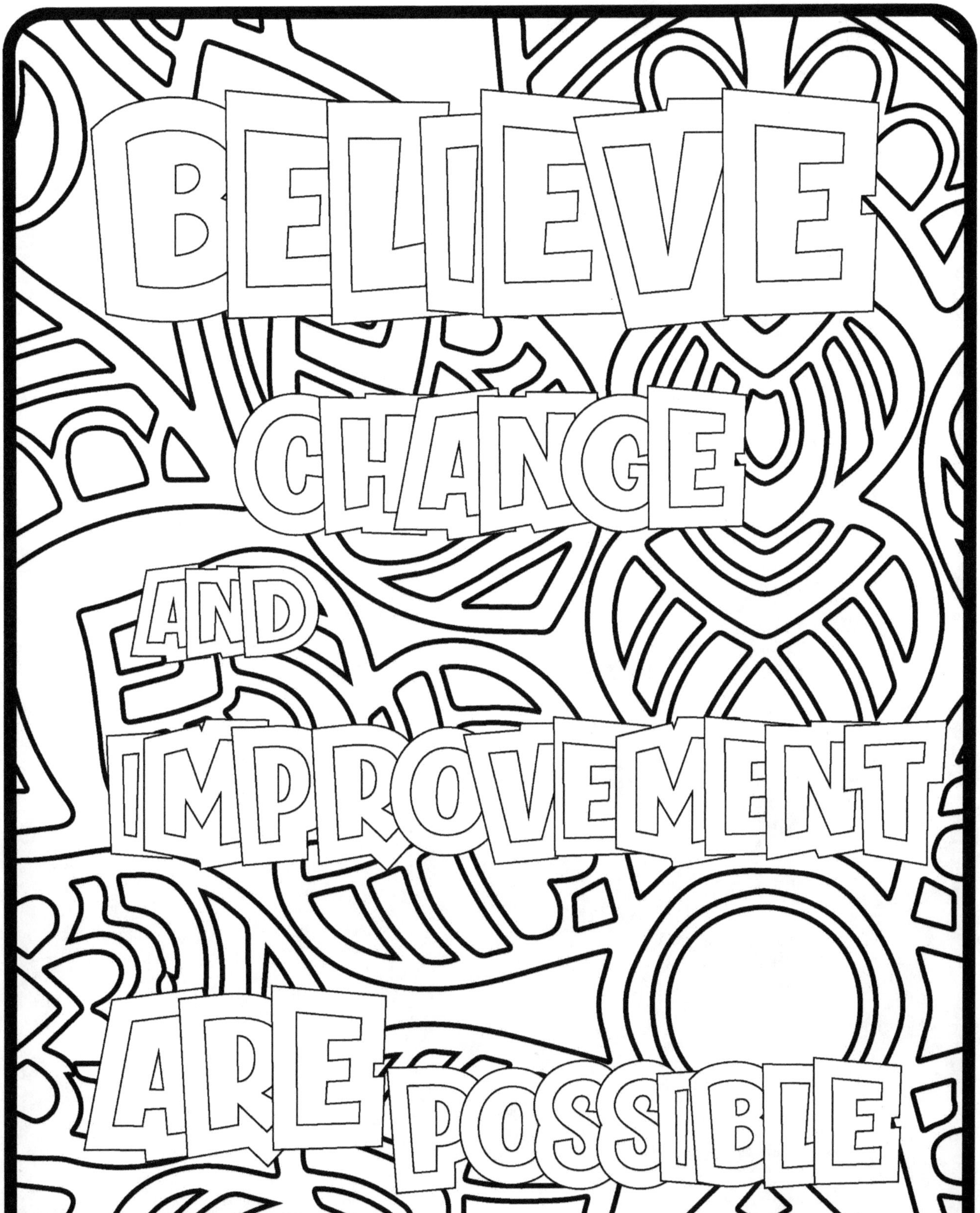
BELIEVE
CHANGE
AND
IMPROVEMENT
ARE POSSIBLE

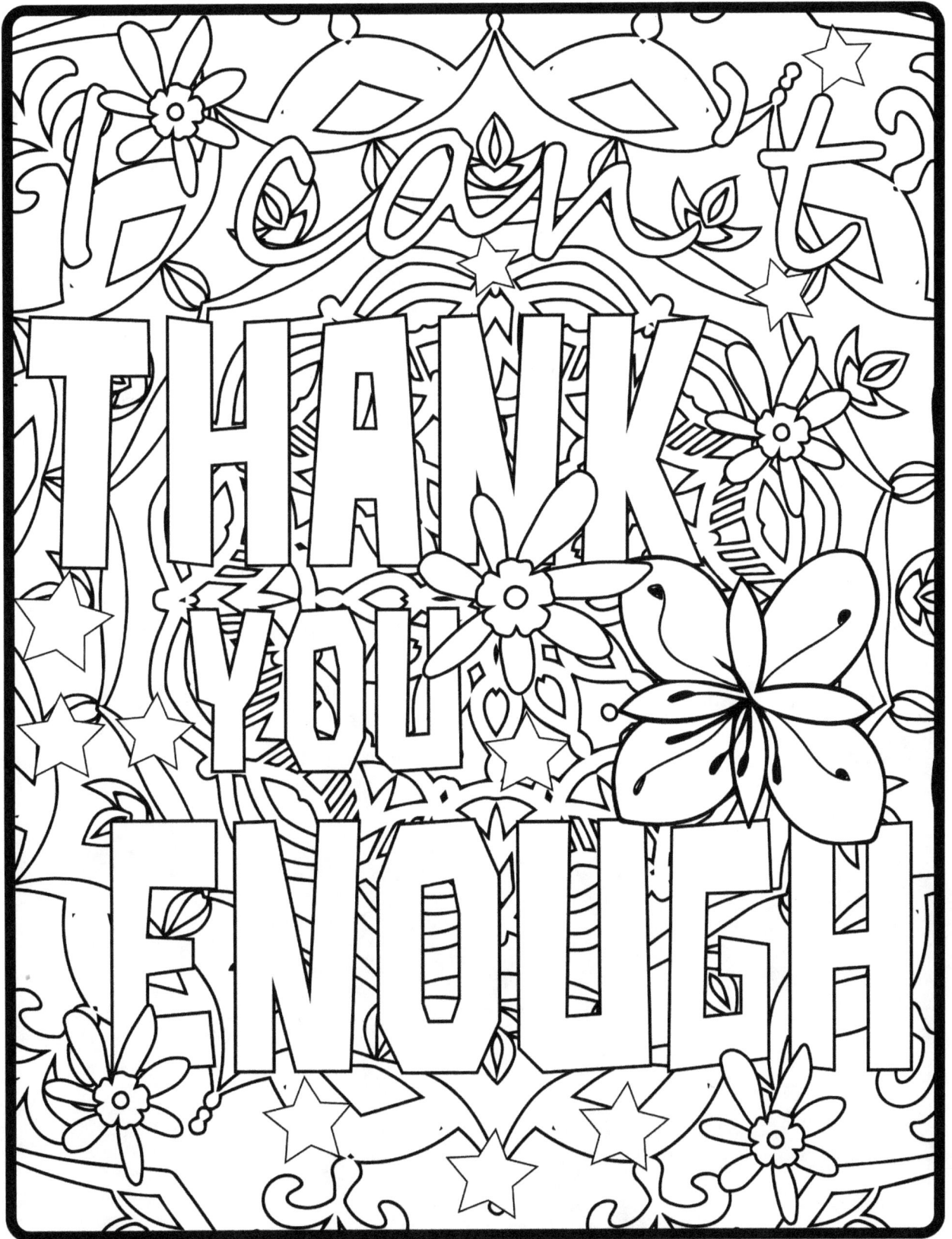

I can't THANK YOU ENOUGH

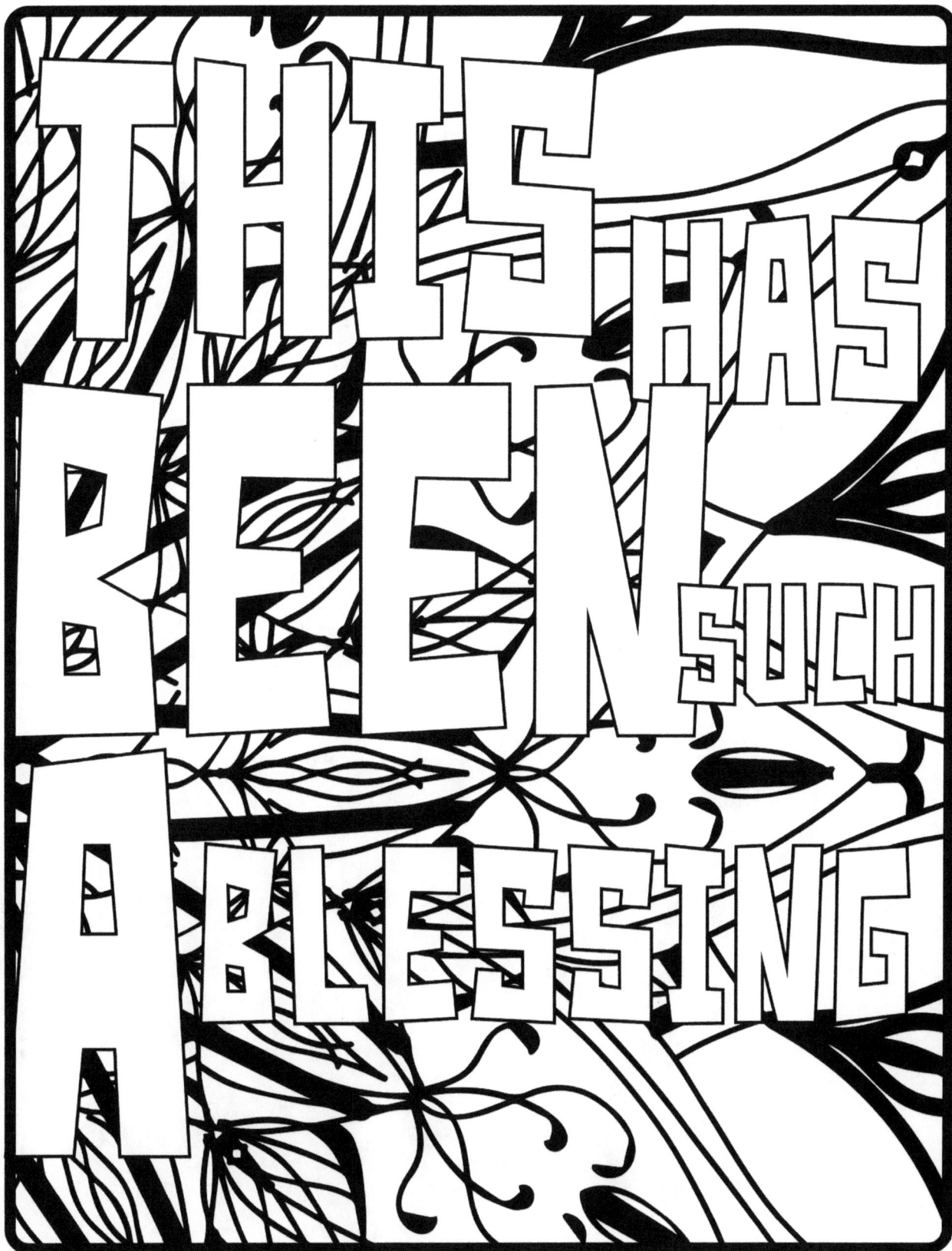

THIS HAS BEEN SUCH A BLESSING

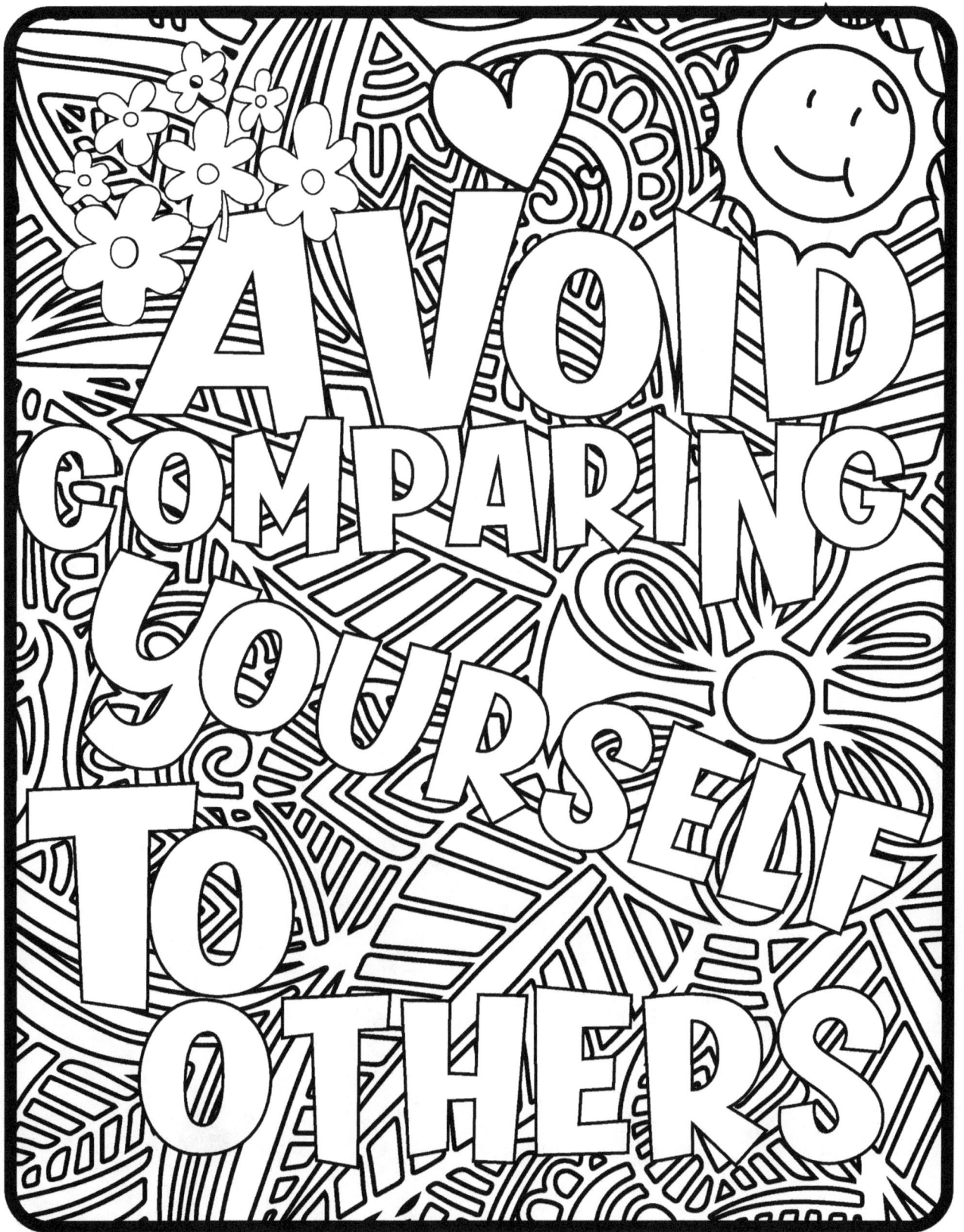

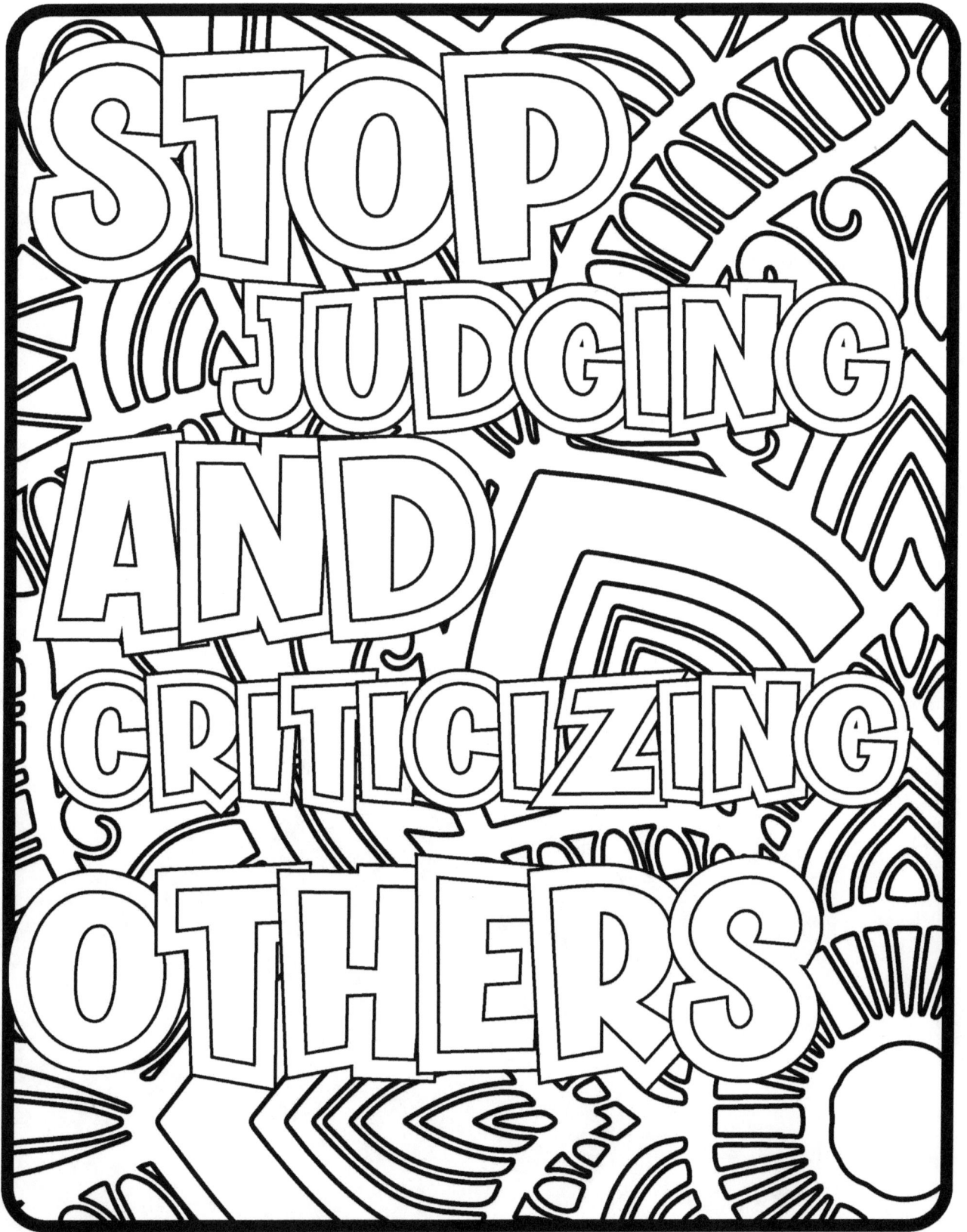

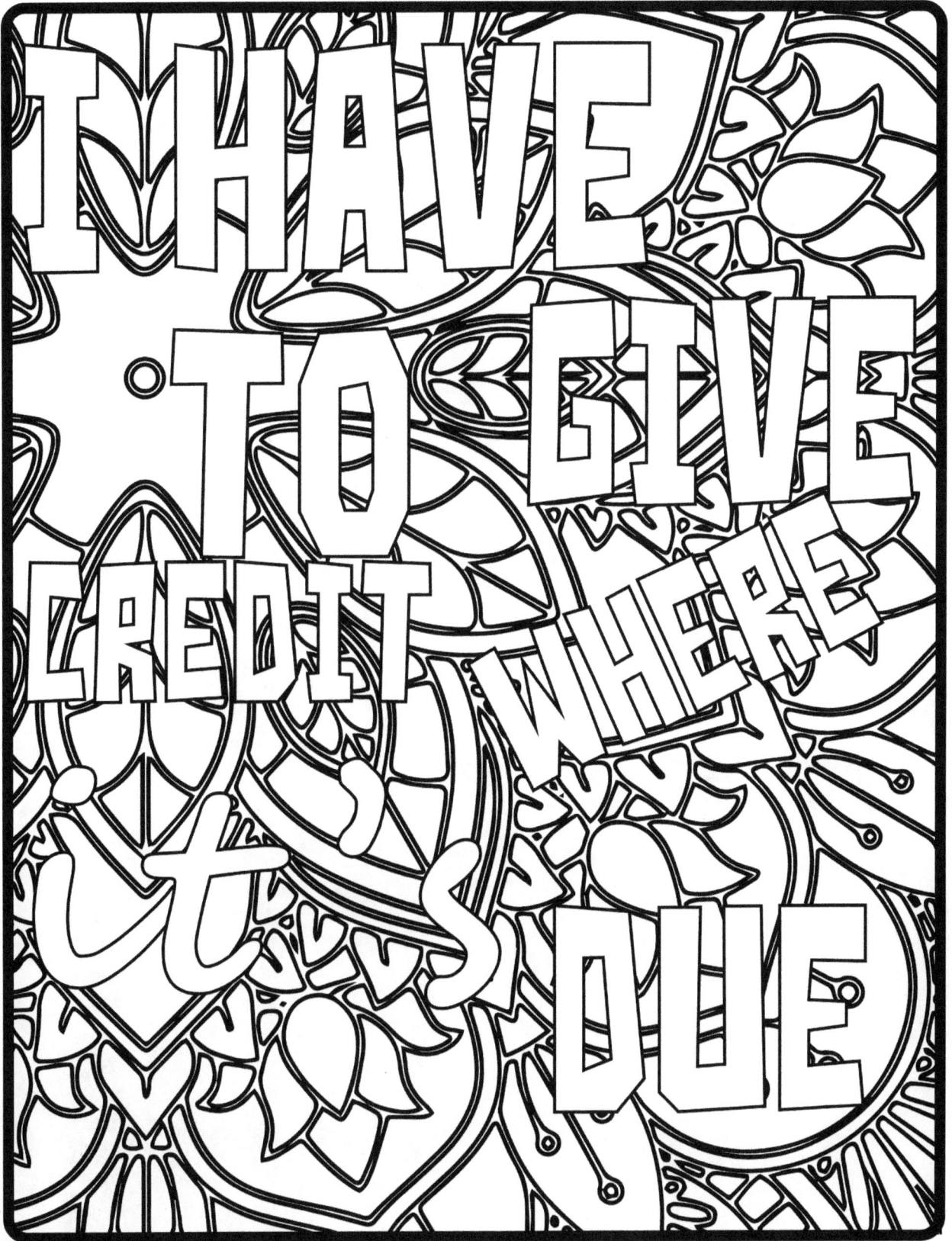

I HAVE TO GIVE CREDIT WHERE IT'S DUE

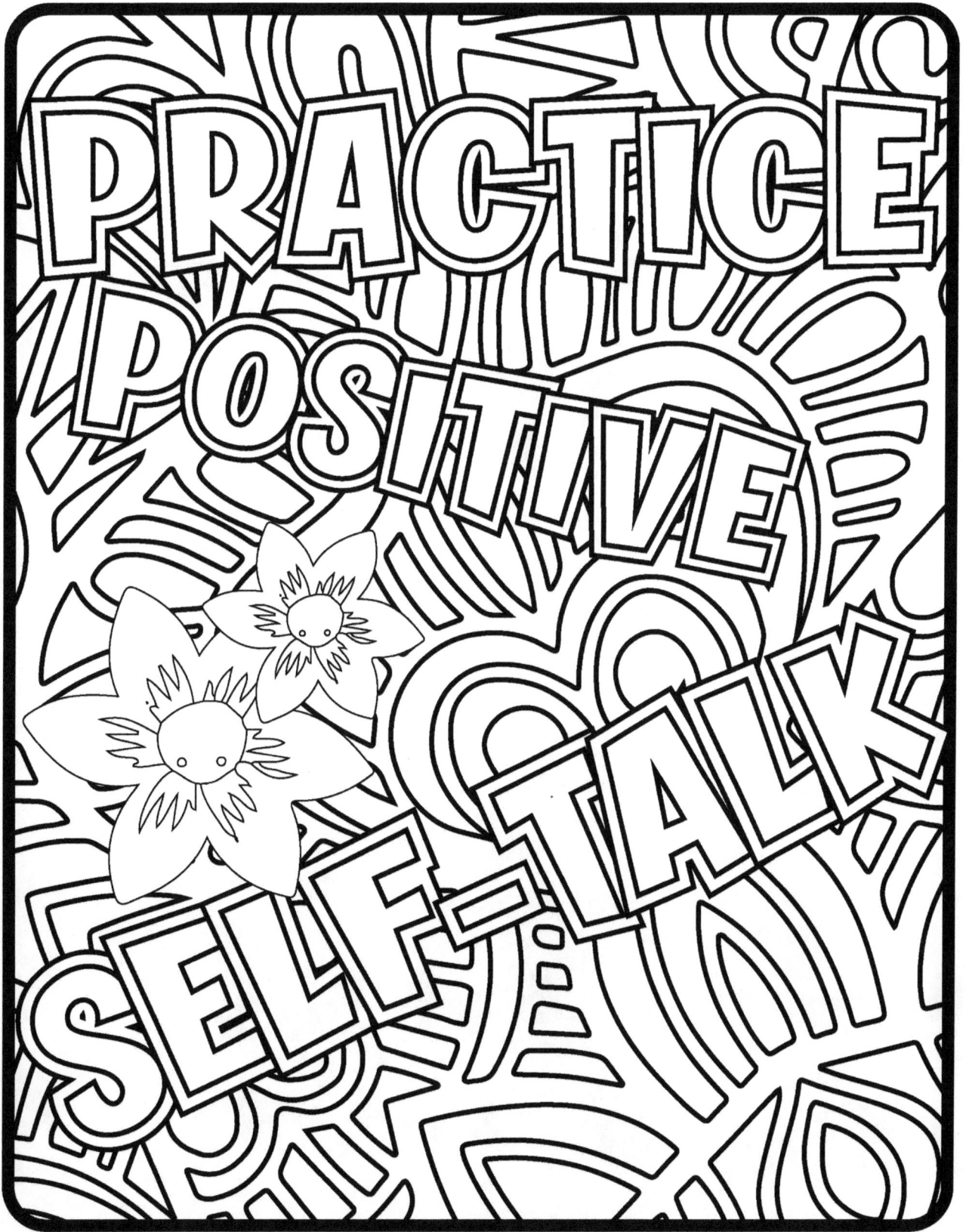

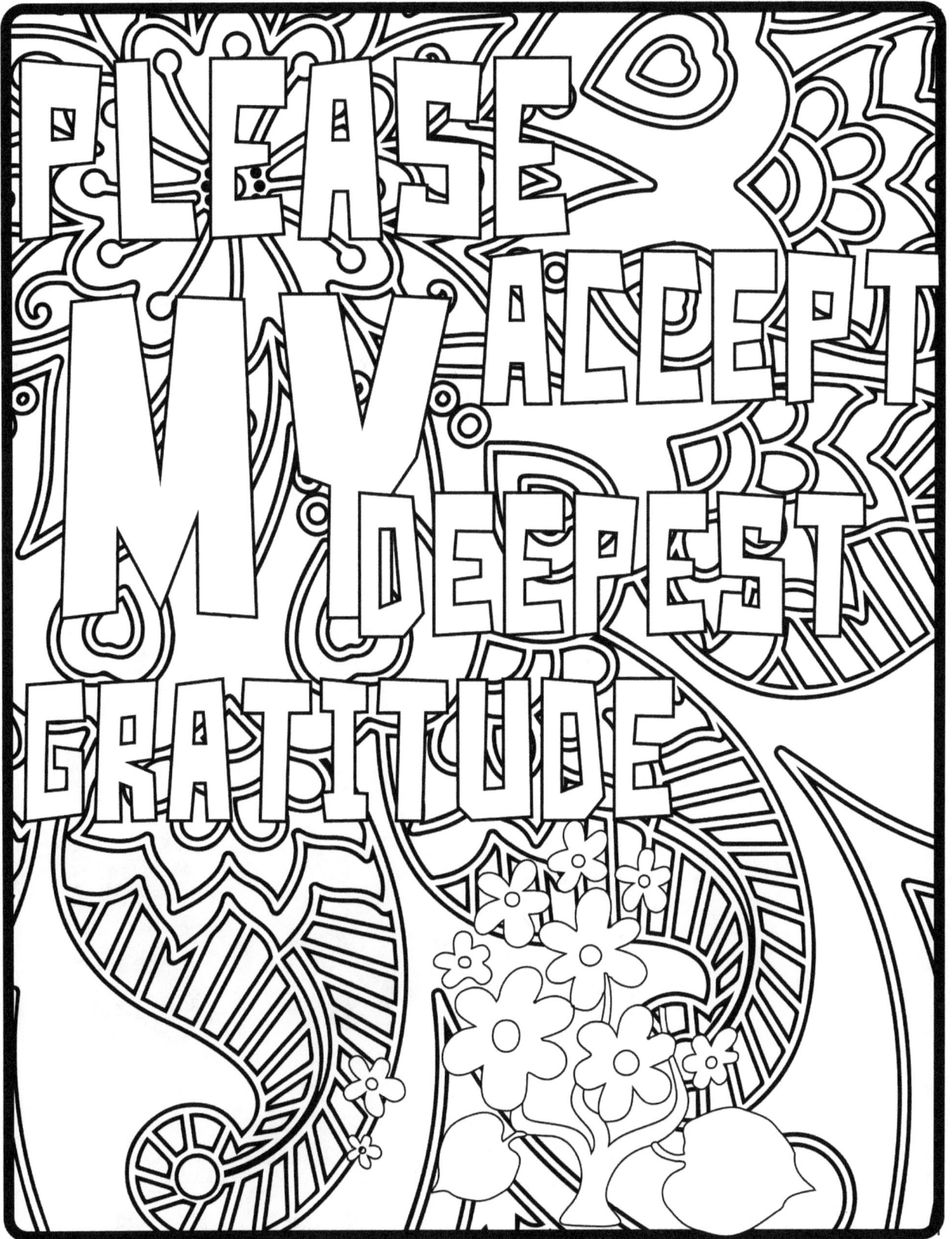

PLEASE ACCEPT MY DEEPEST GRATITUDE

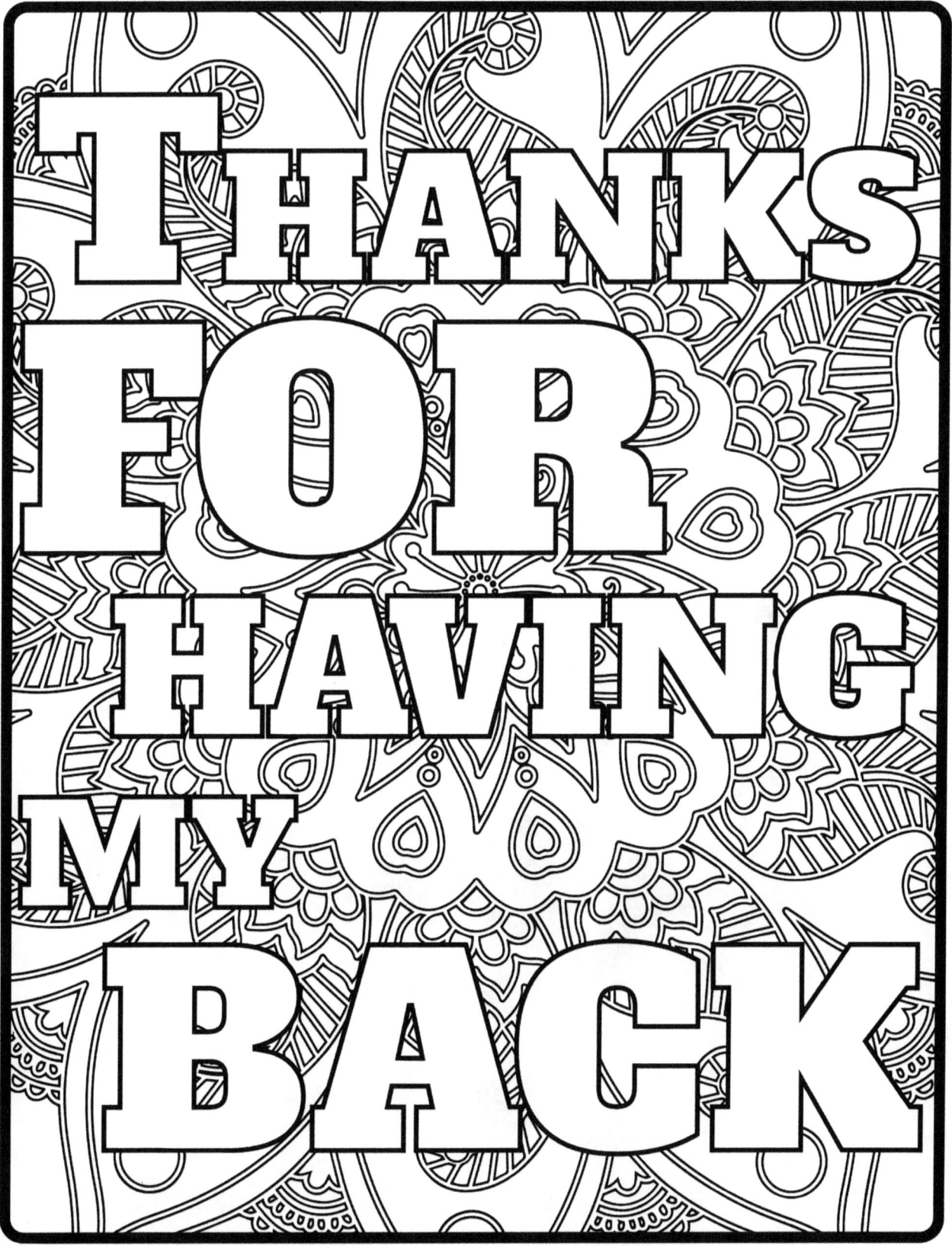

THANKS FOR HAVING MY BACK

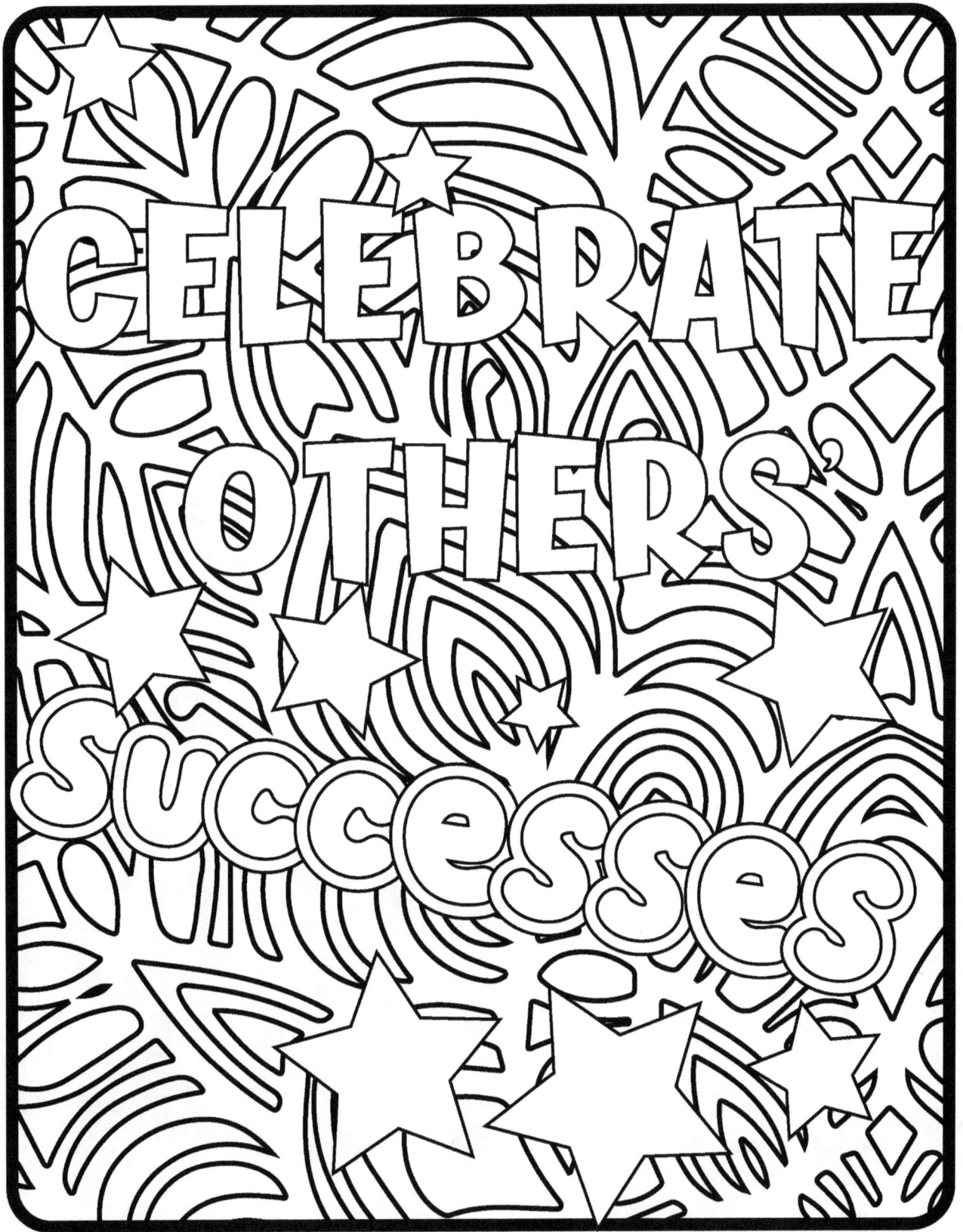

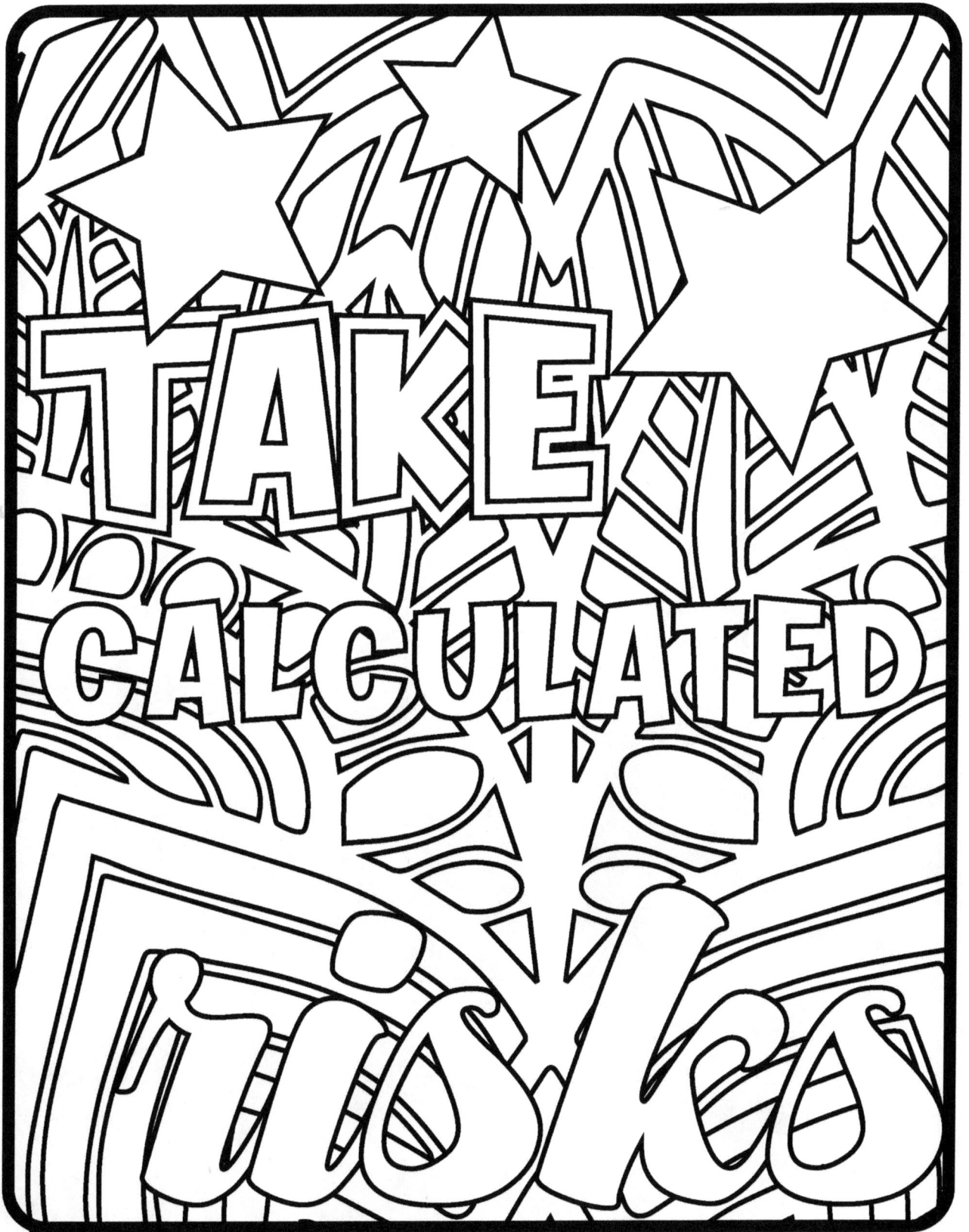

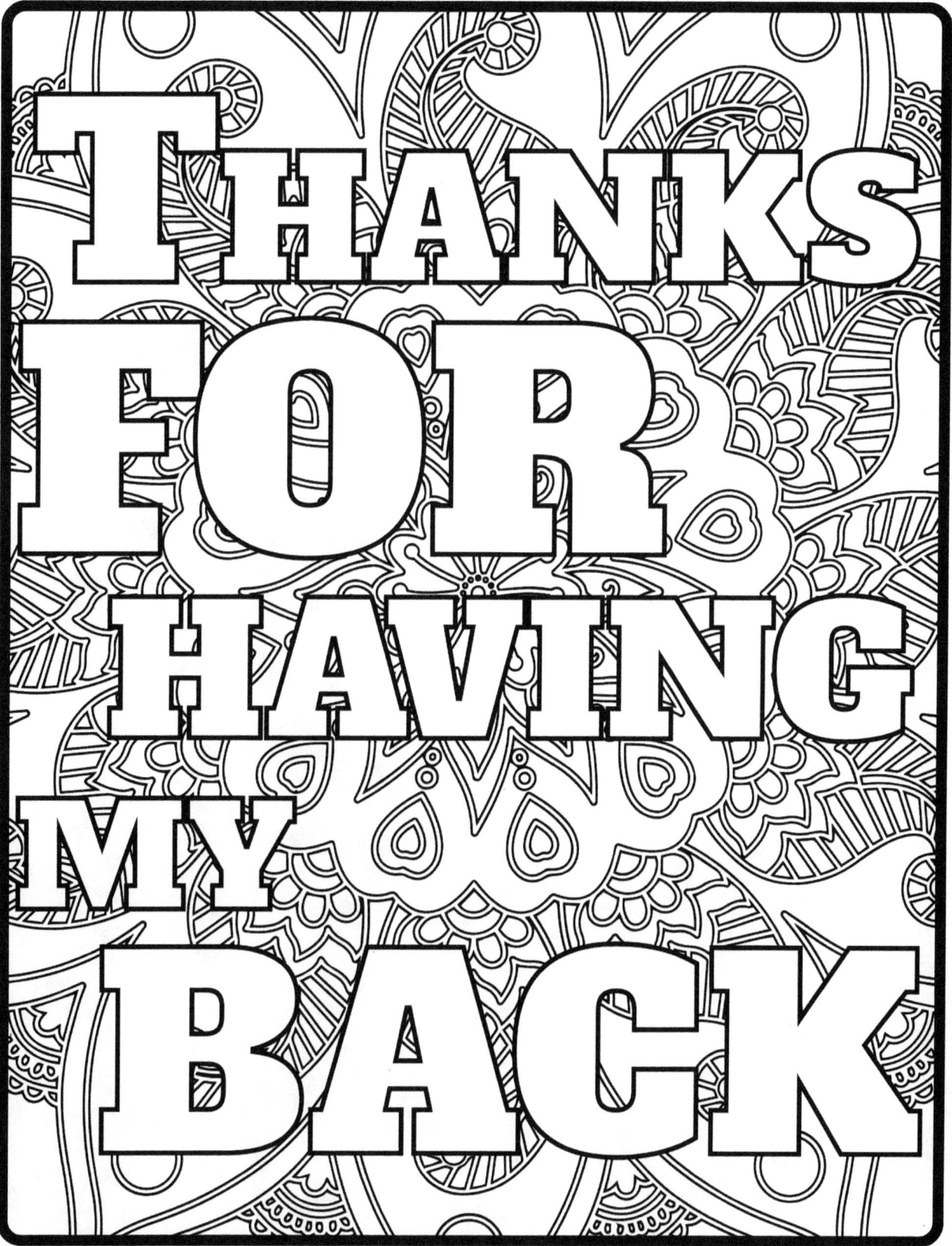

THANKS FOR HAVING MY BACK

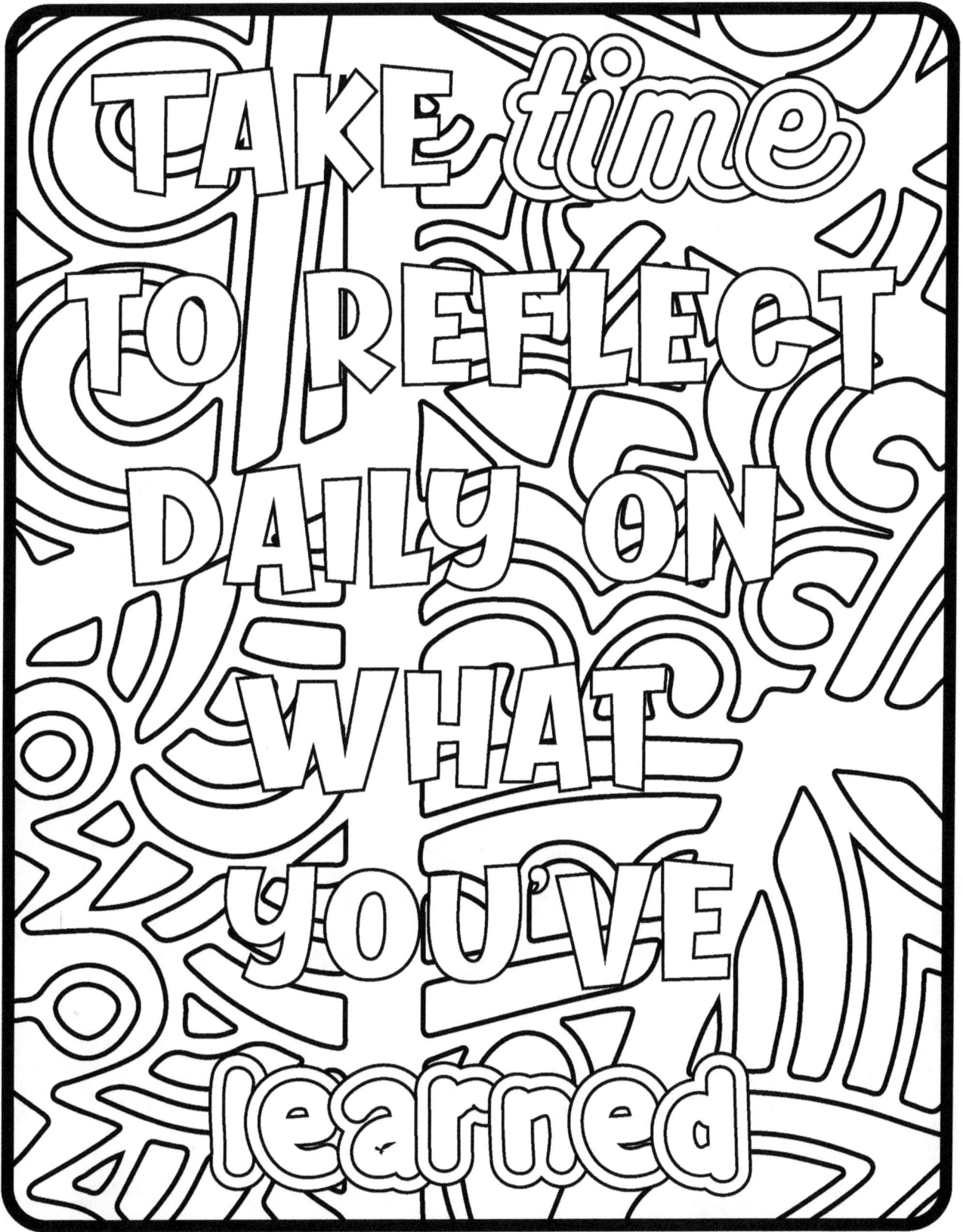

TAKE time TO REFLECT DAILY ON WHAT YOU'VE learned

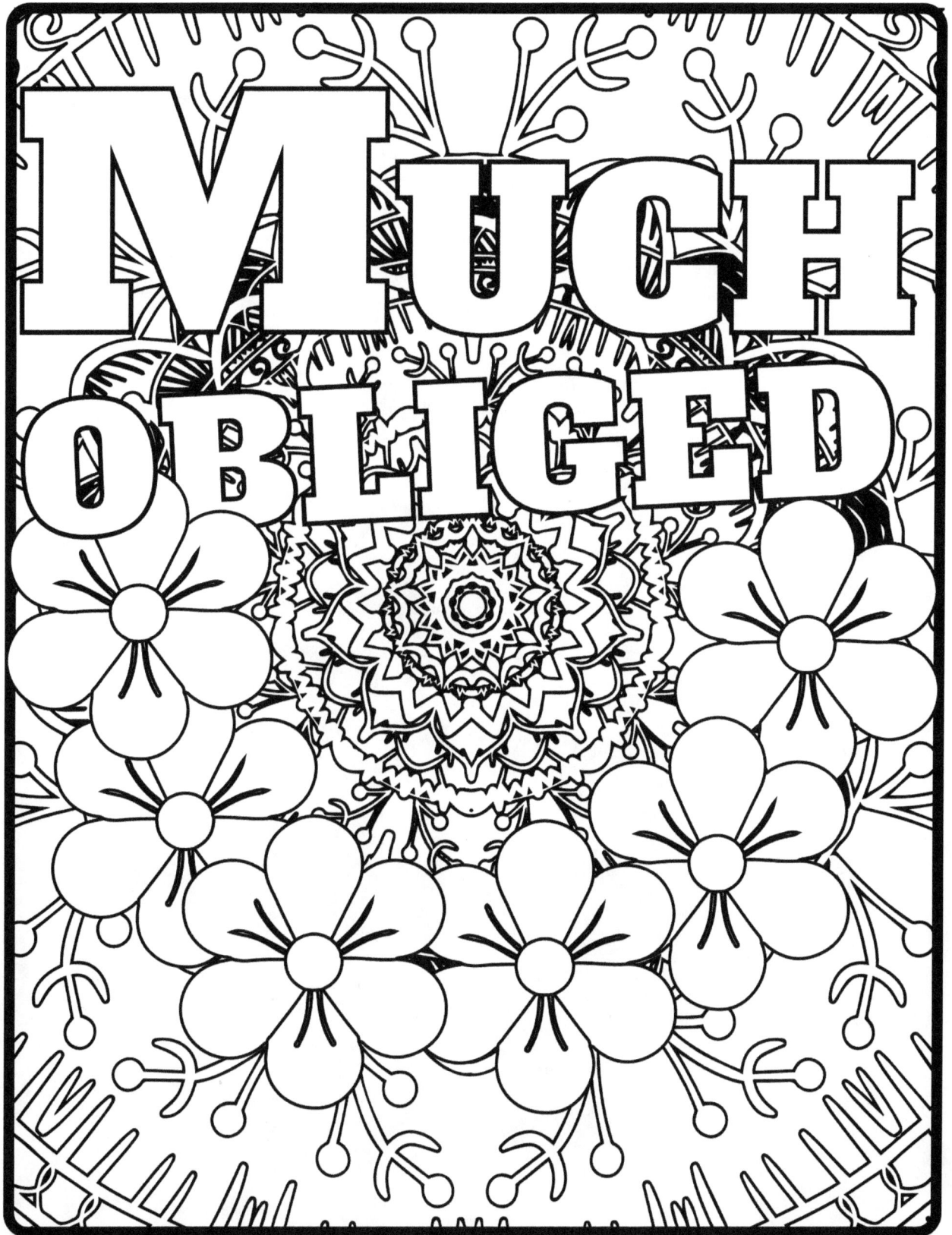

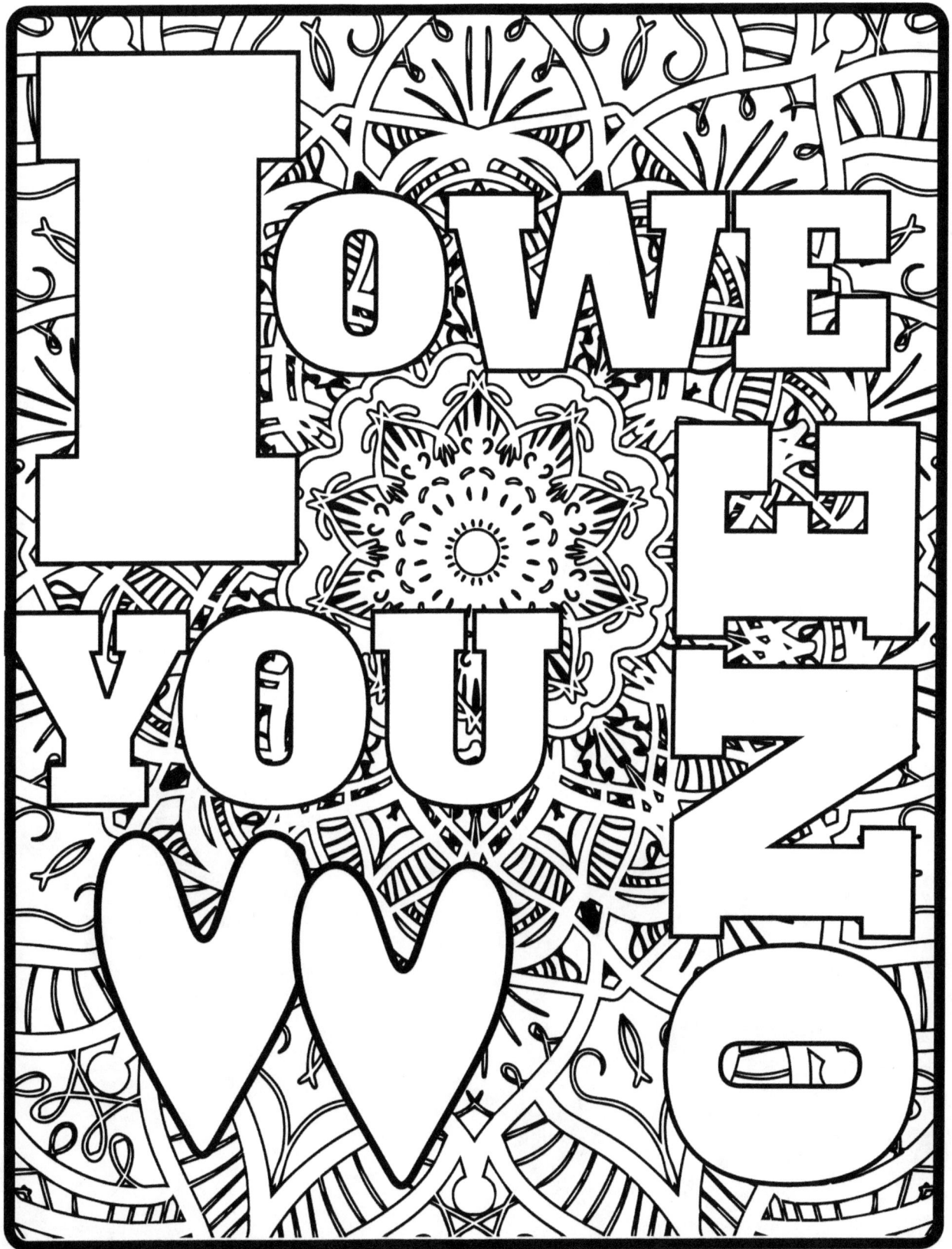

I OWE YOU NO ♥♥

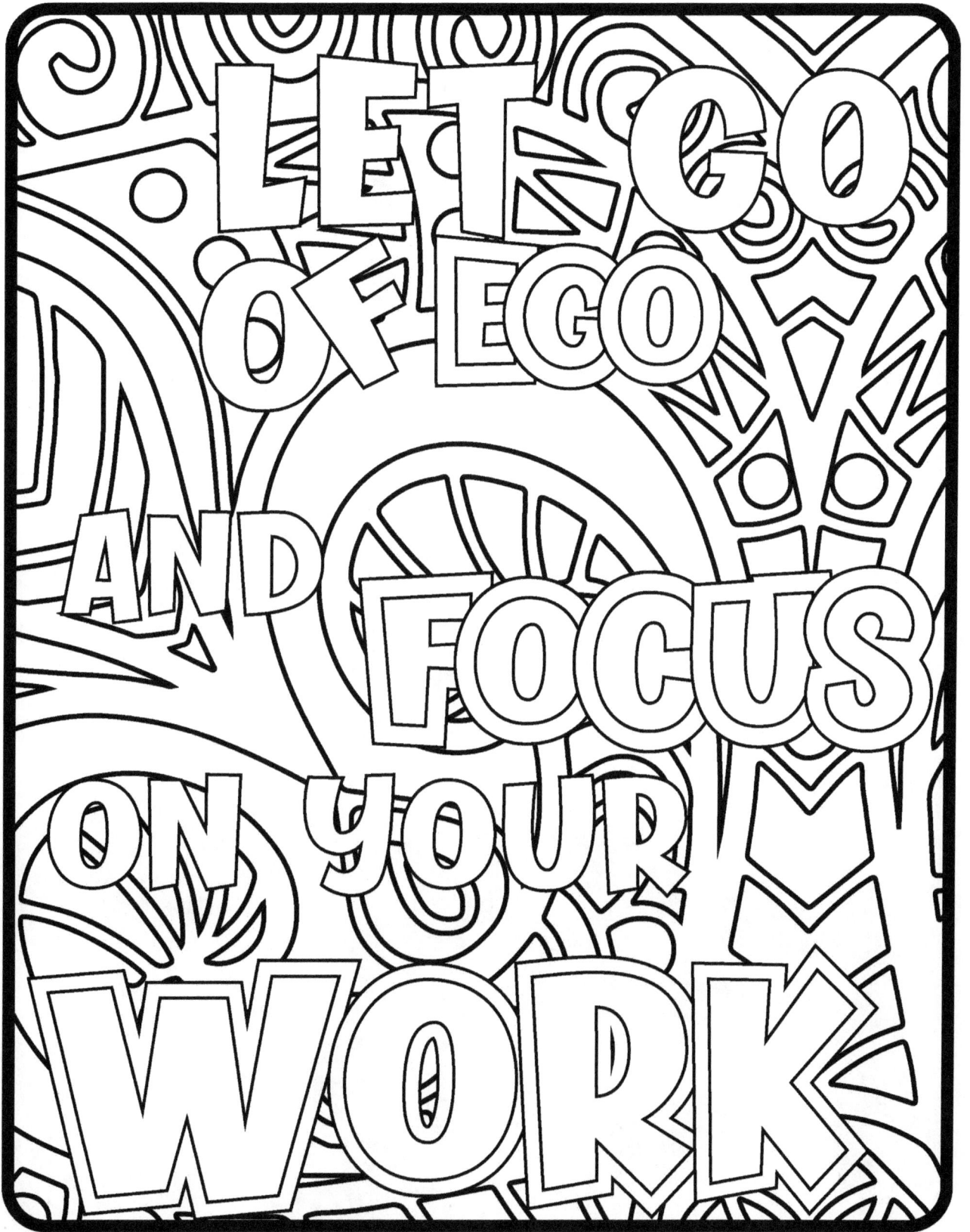

LET GO OF EGO AND FOCUS ON YOUR WORK

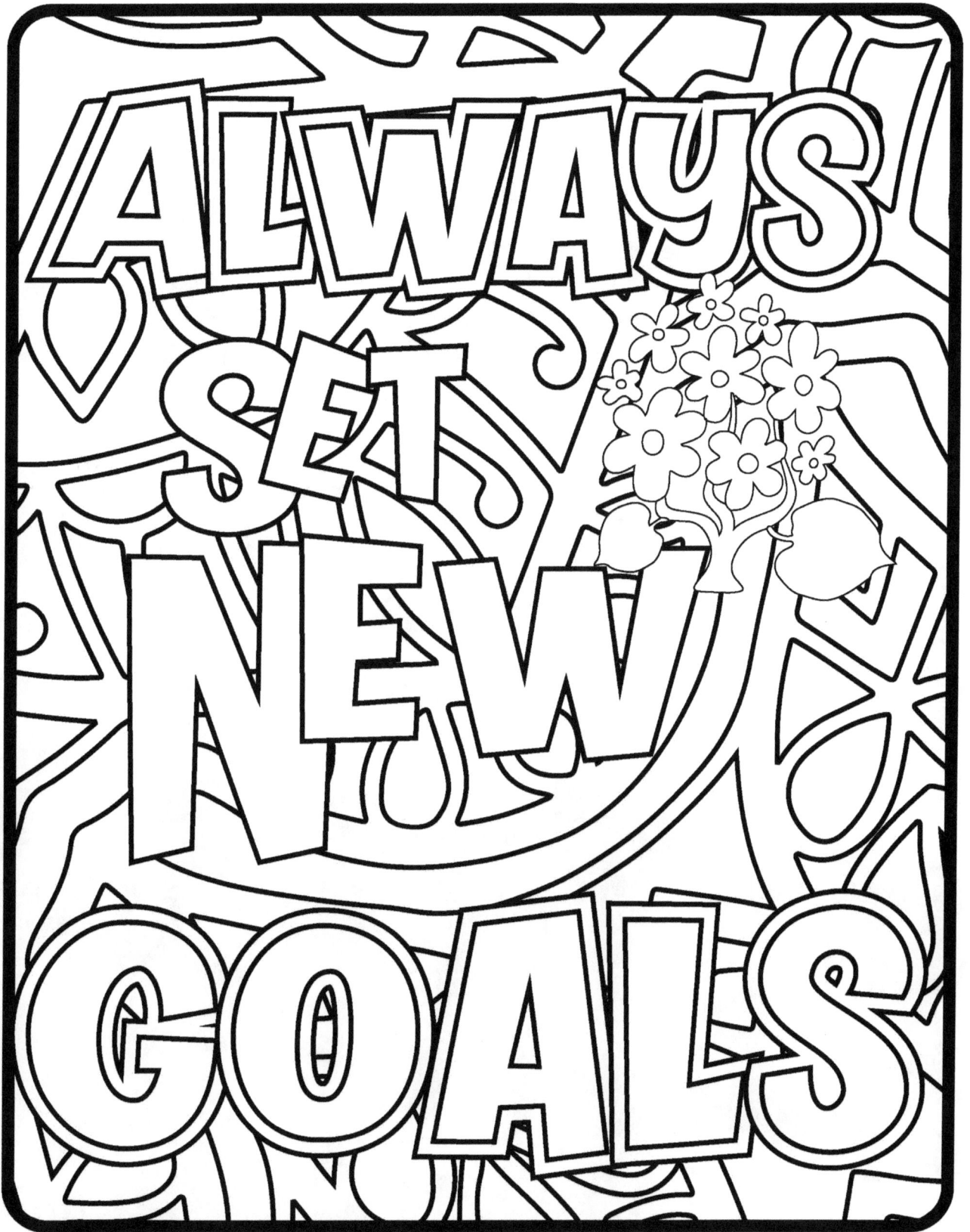

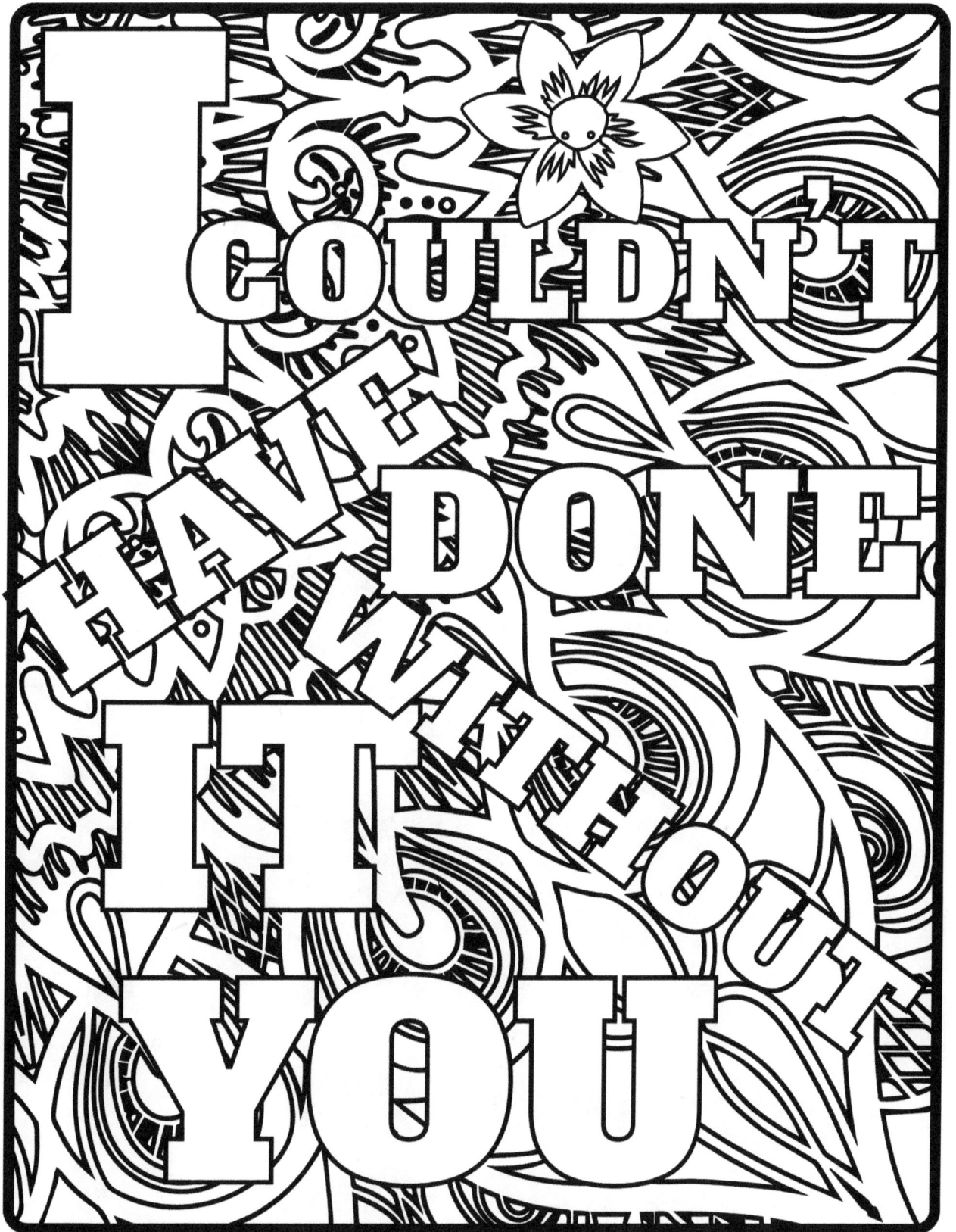

I COULDN'T HAVE DONE IT WITHOUT YOU

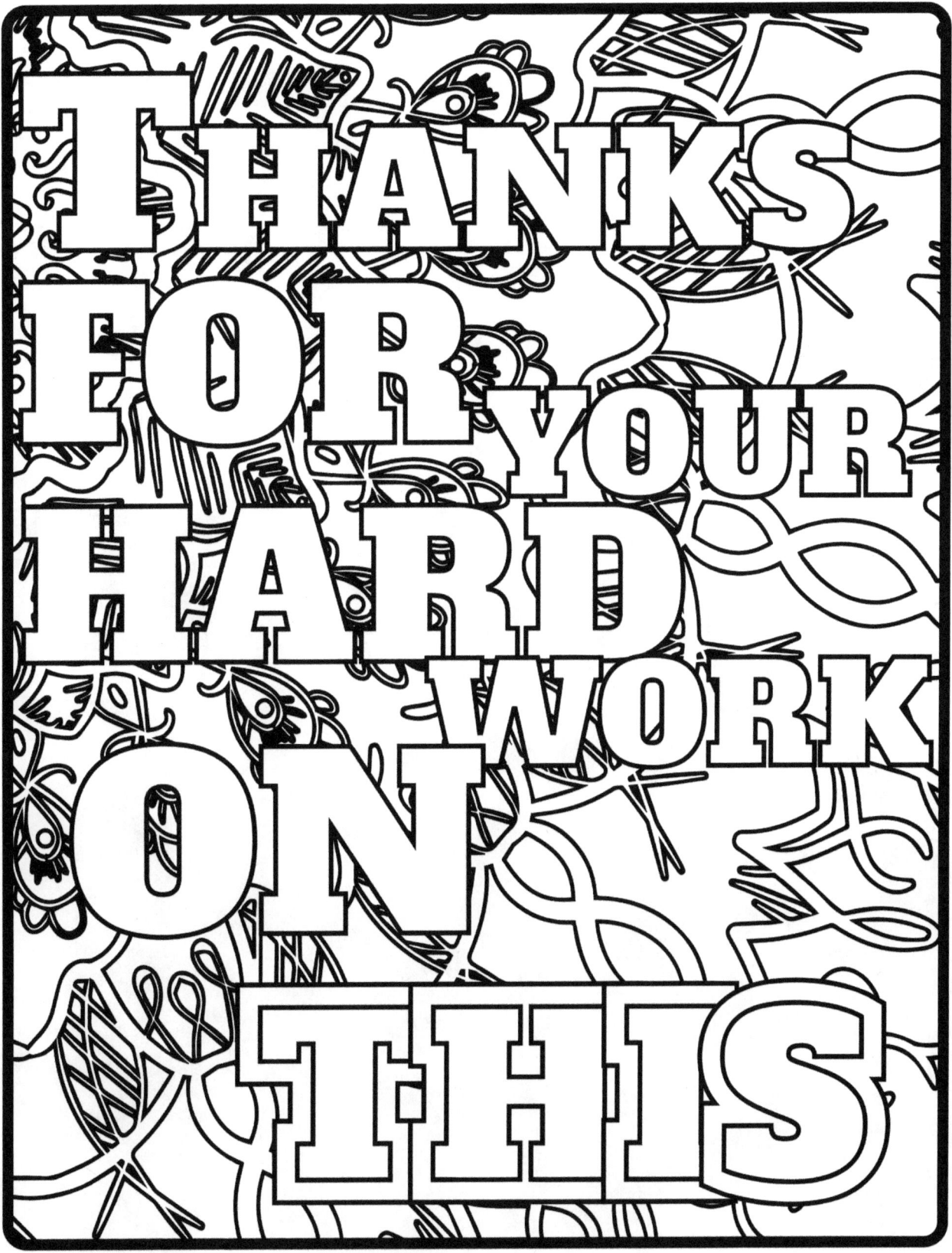

THANKS FOR YOUR HARD WORK ON THIS

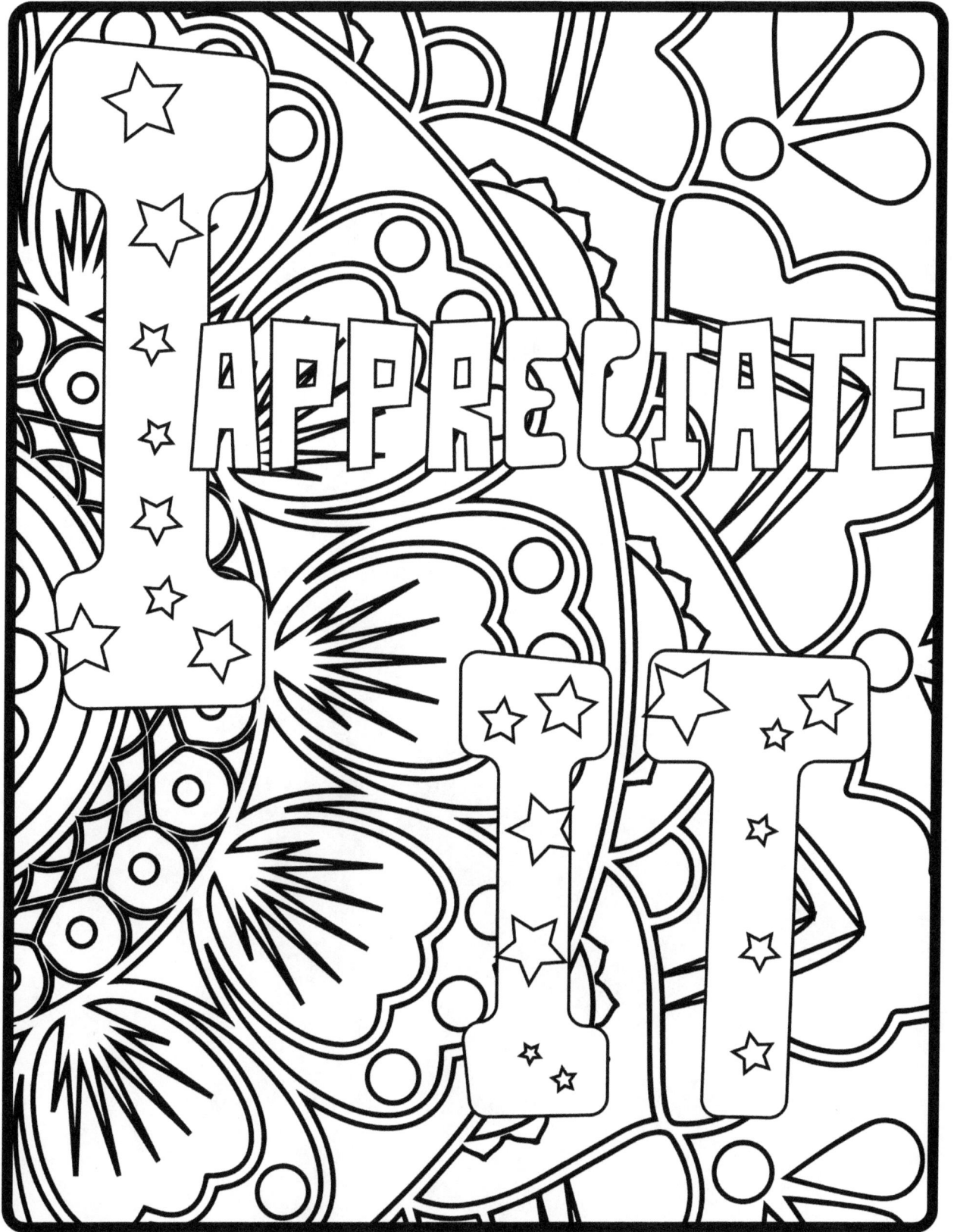

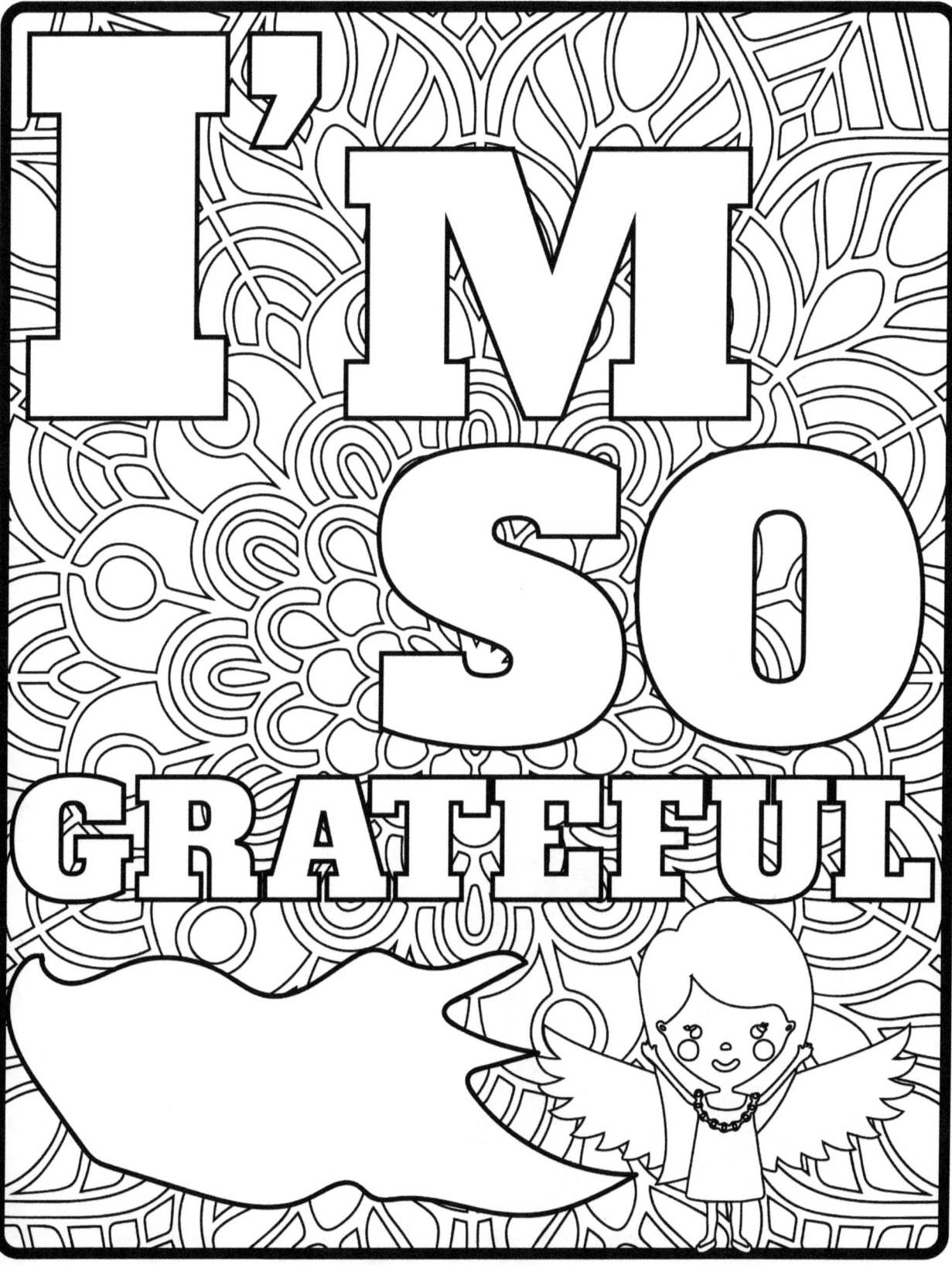

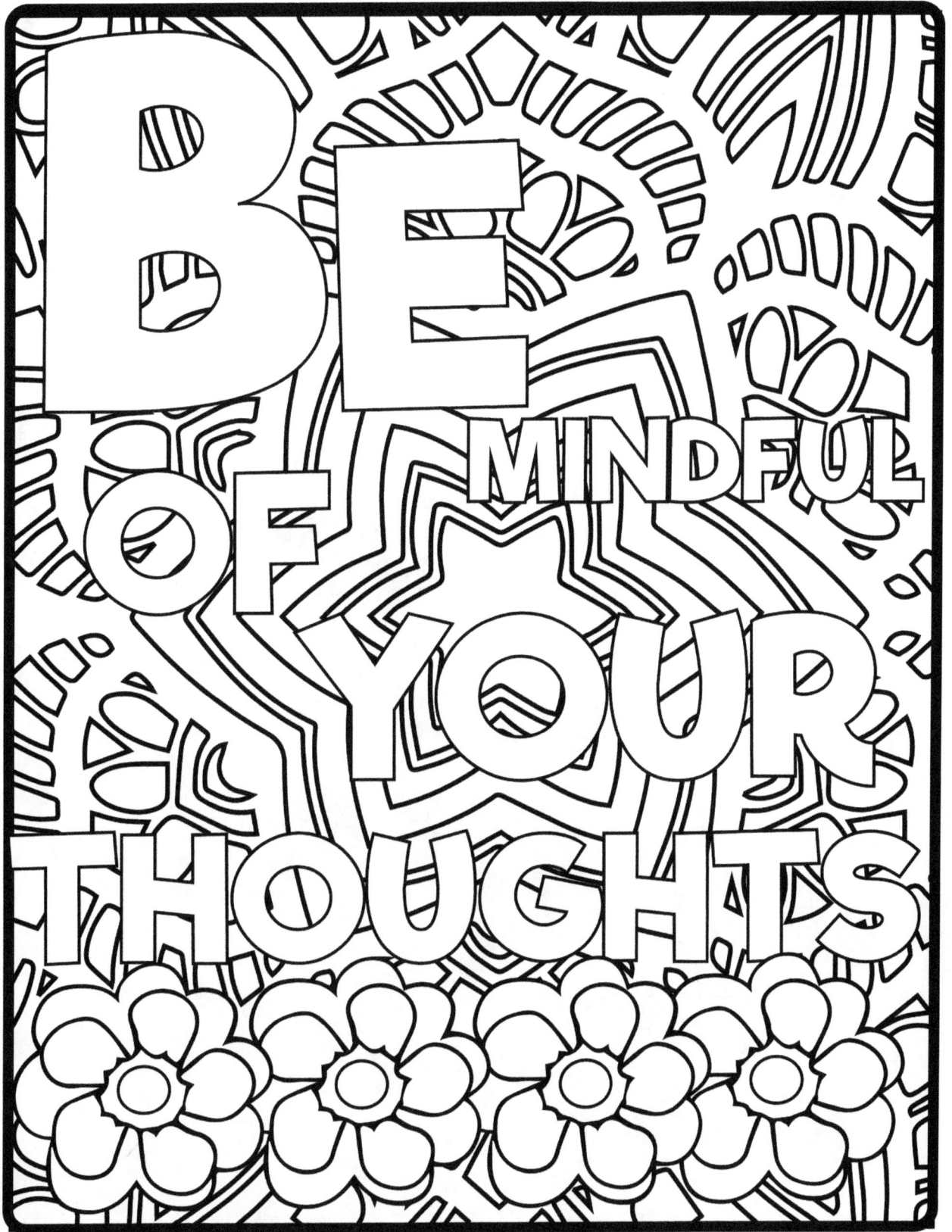

BE MINDFUL OF YOUR THOUGHTS

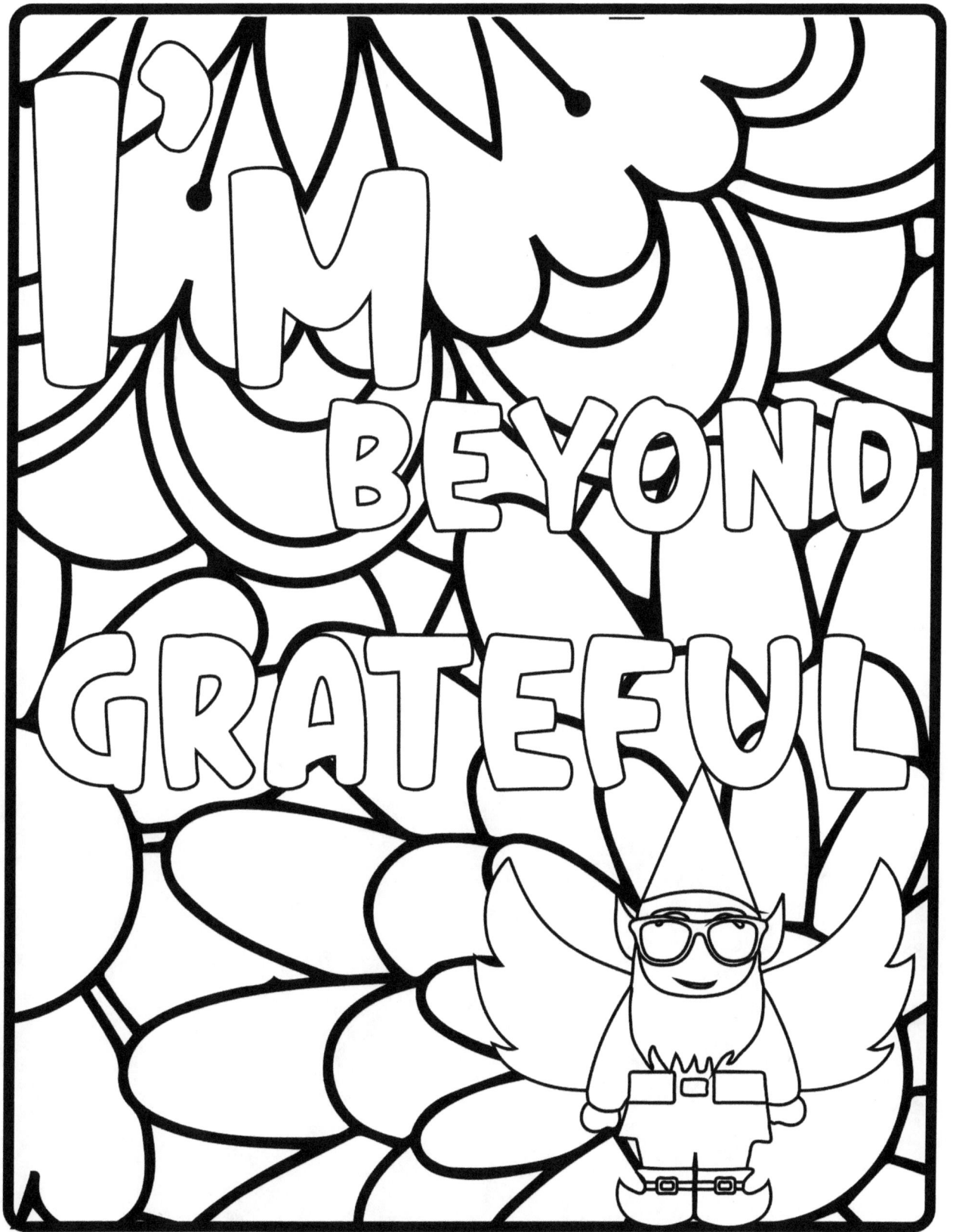

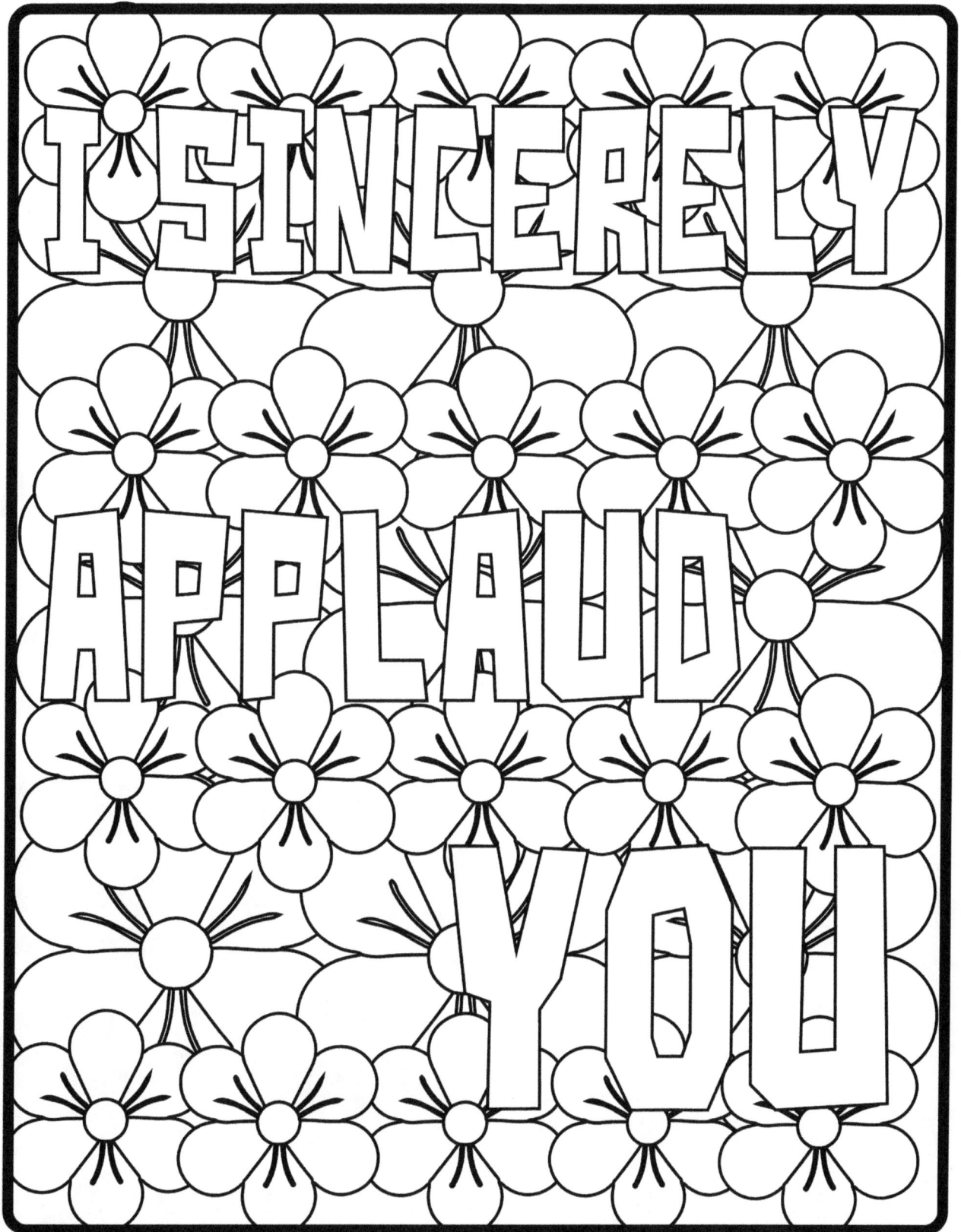

I SINCERELY APPLAUD YOU

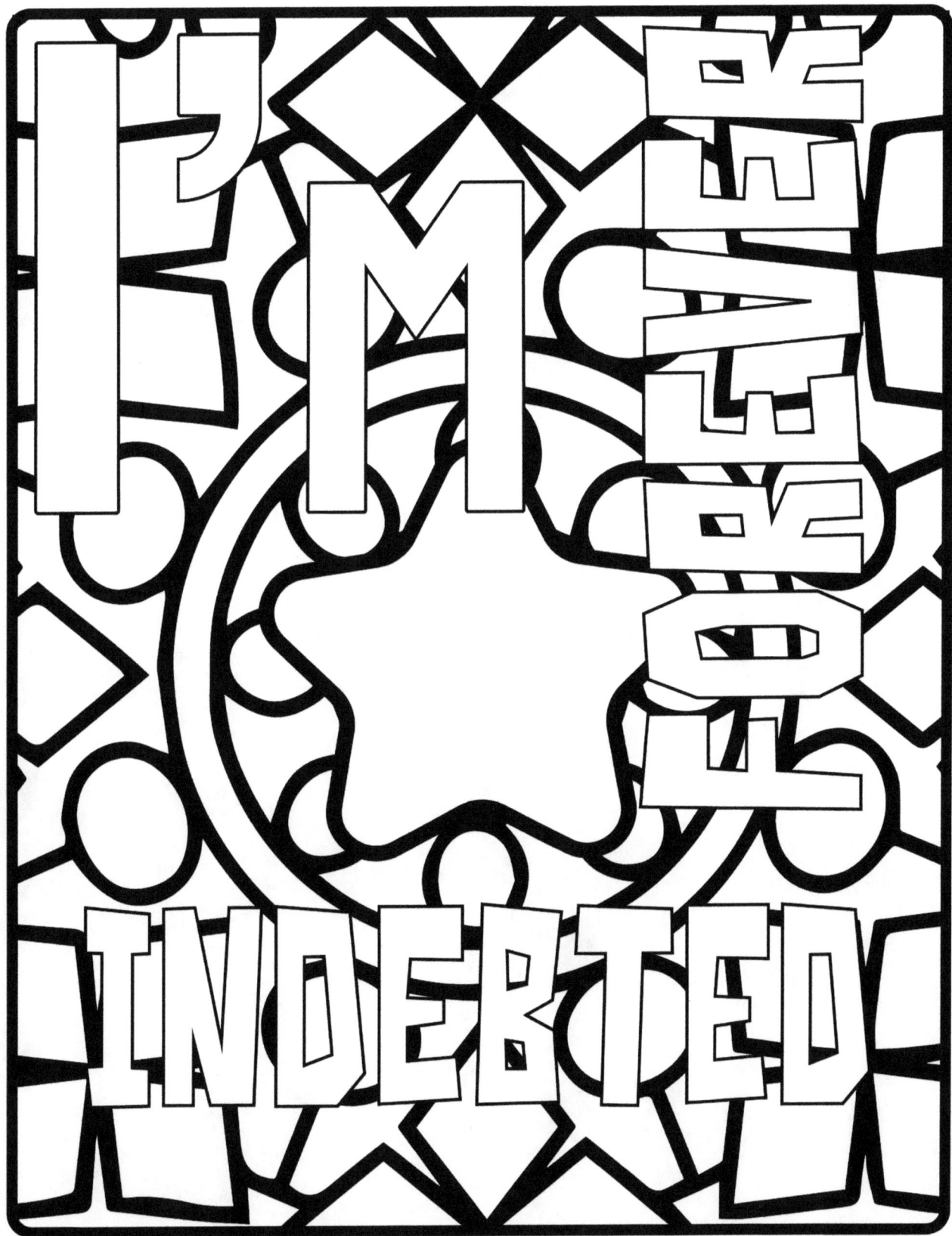

I'M FOREVER INDEBTED

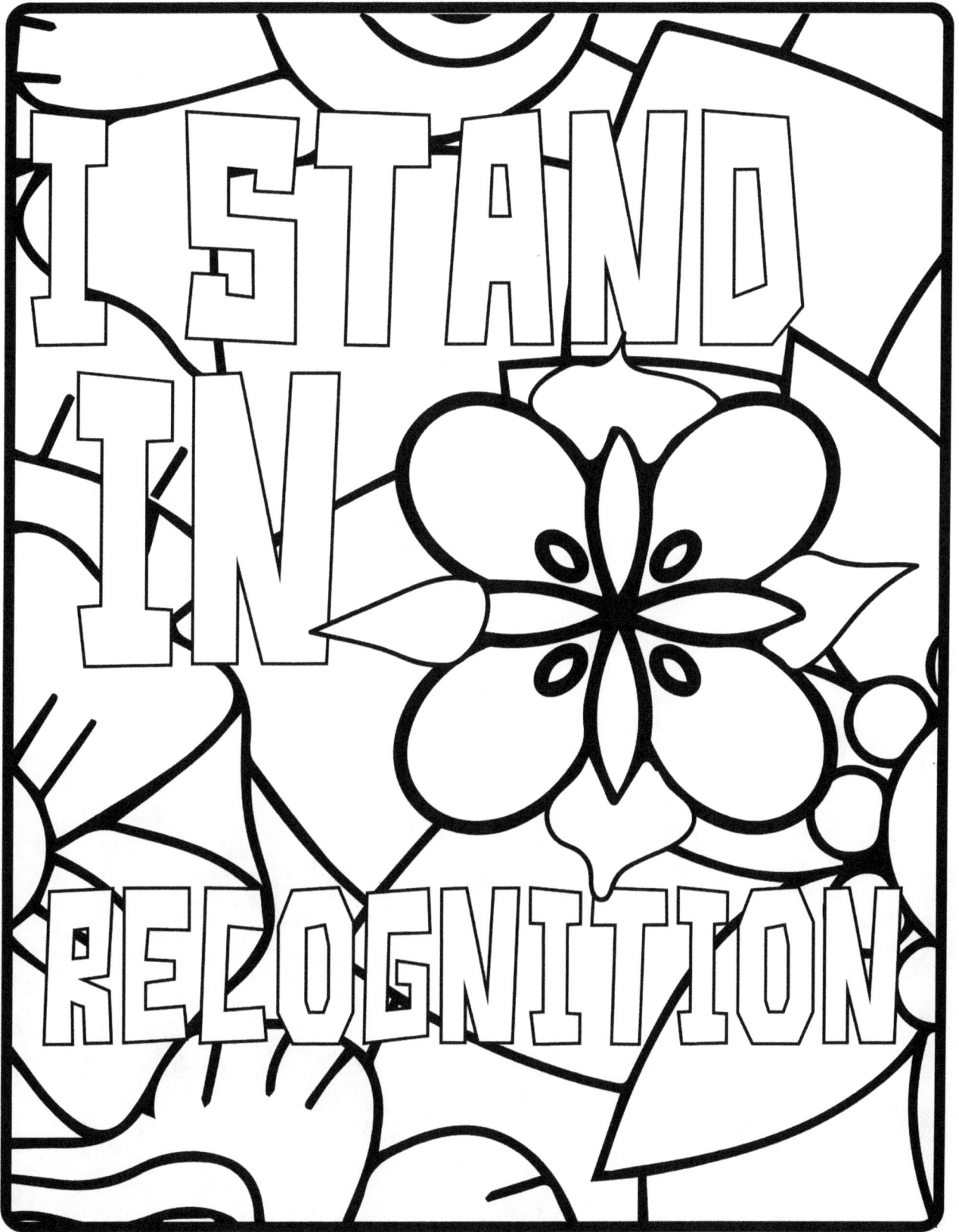

I STAND IN RECOGNITION

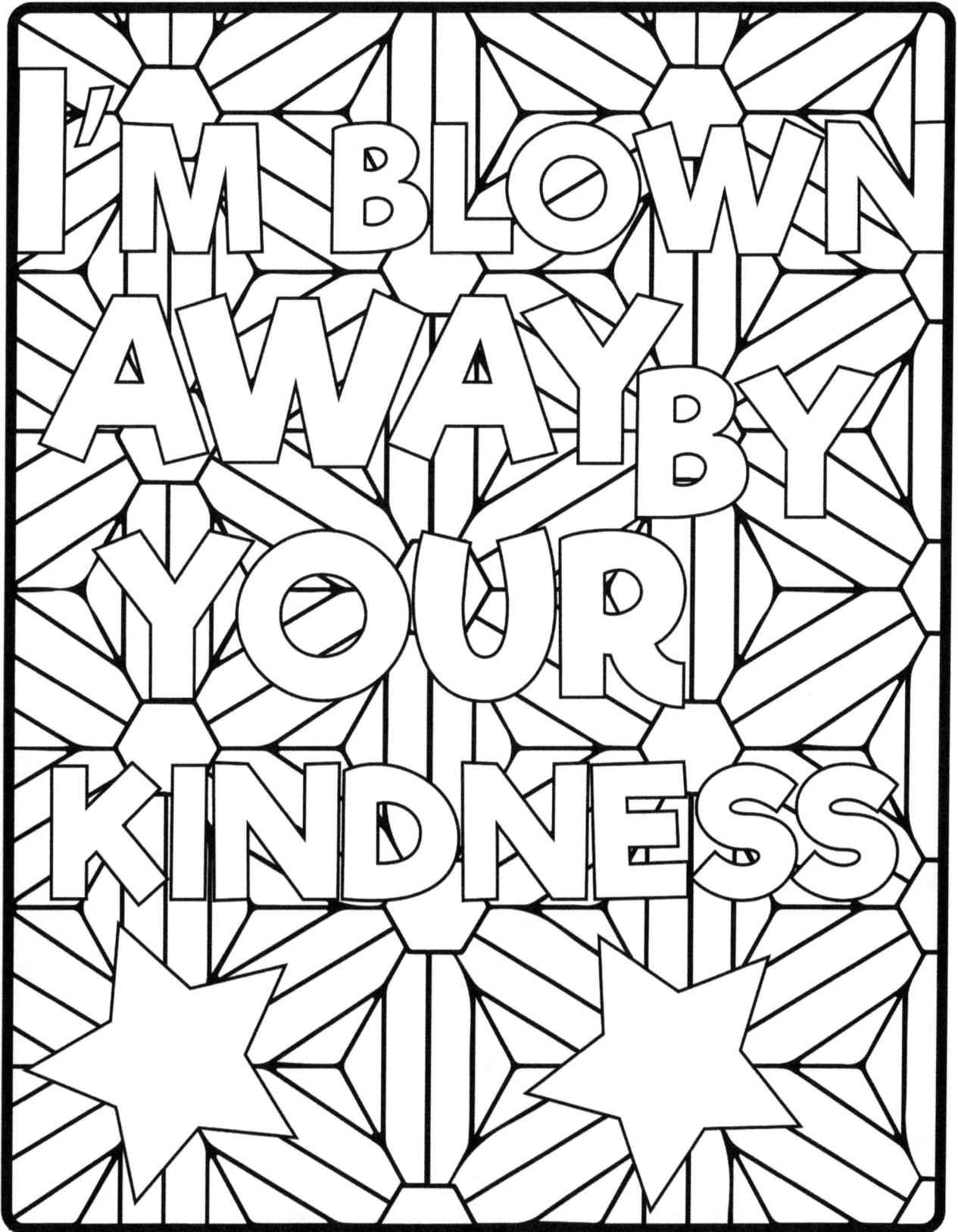

I'M BLOWN AWAY BY YOUR KINDNESS

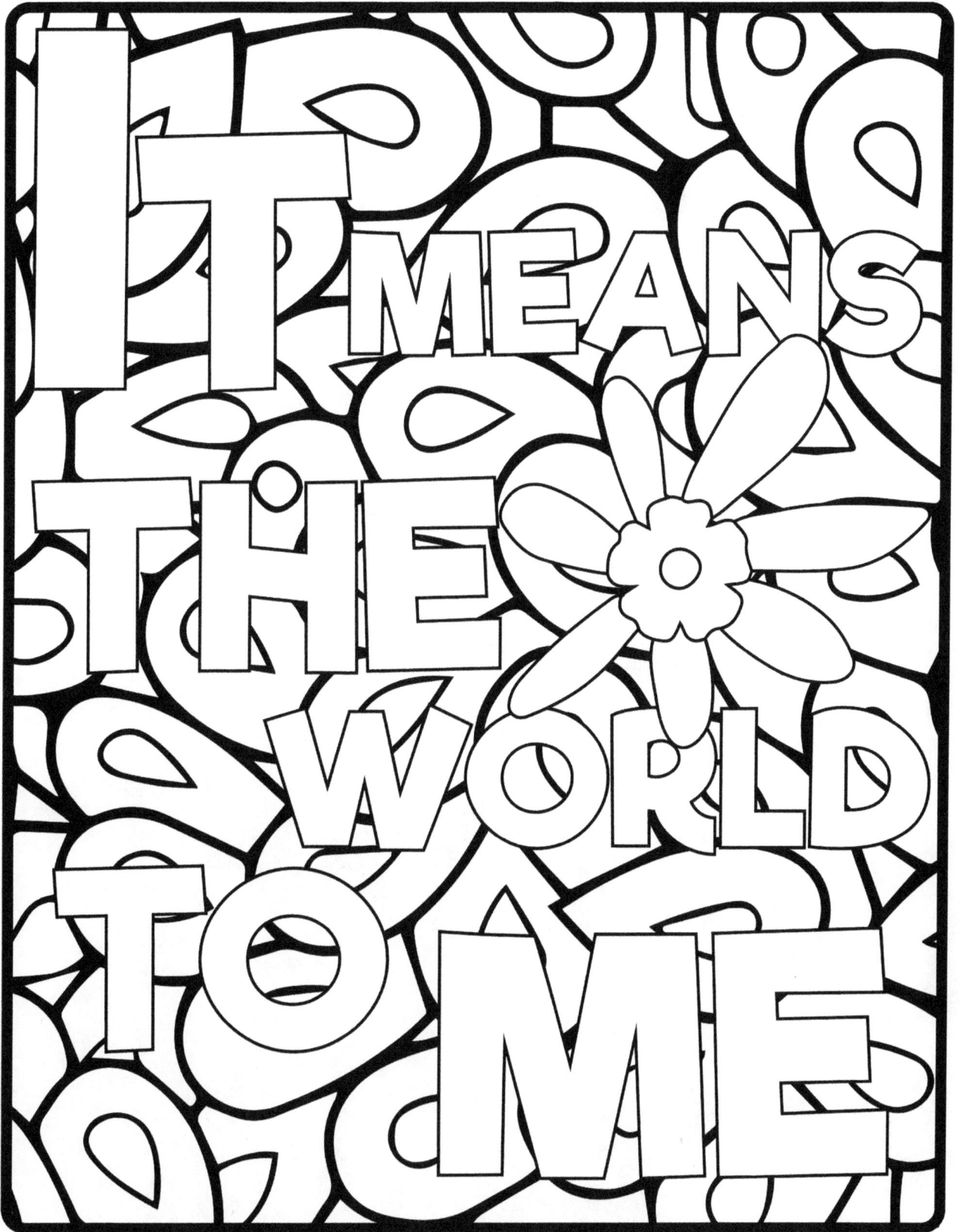
IT MEANS THE WORLD TO ME

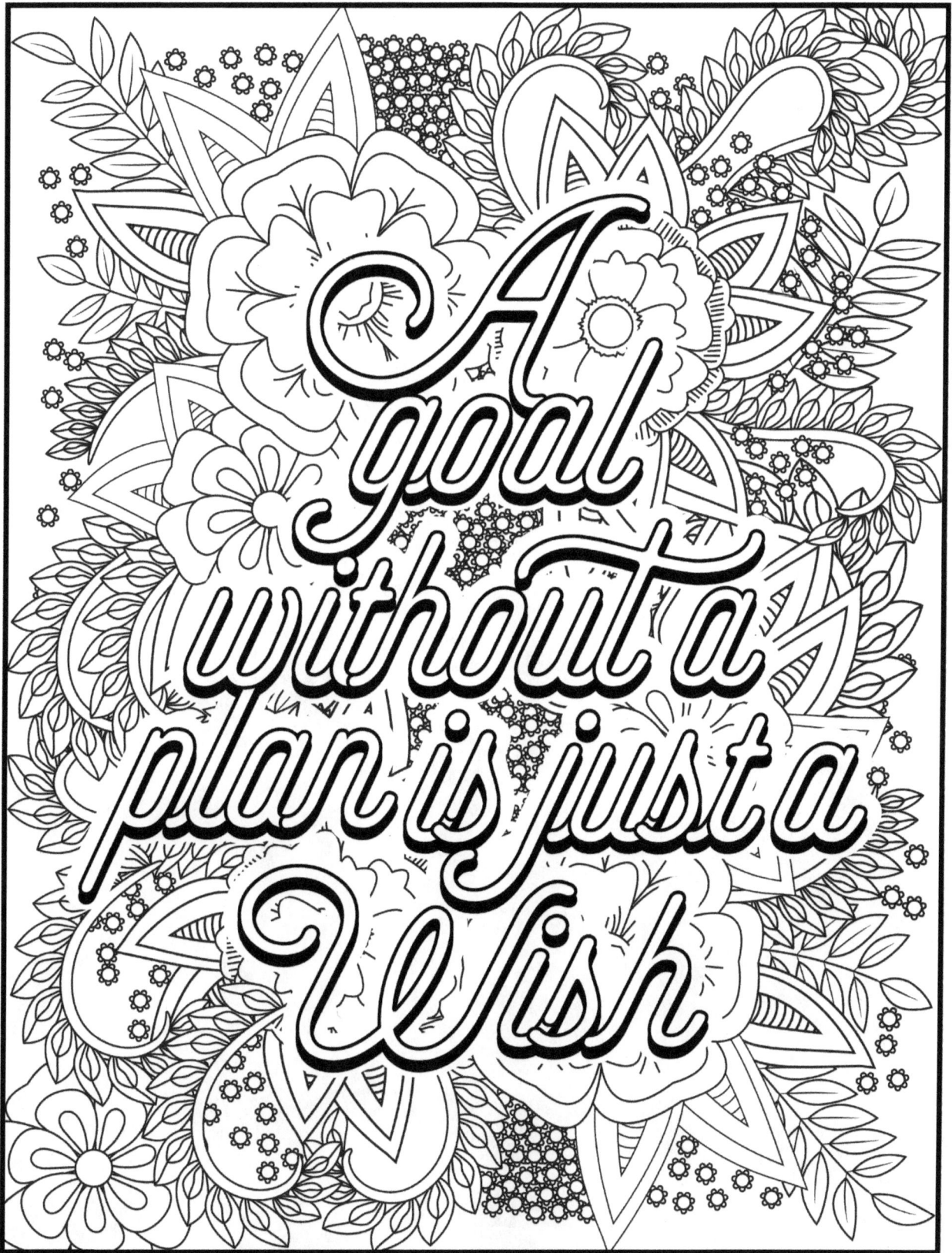

A goal without a plan is just a Wish

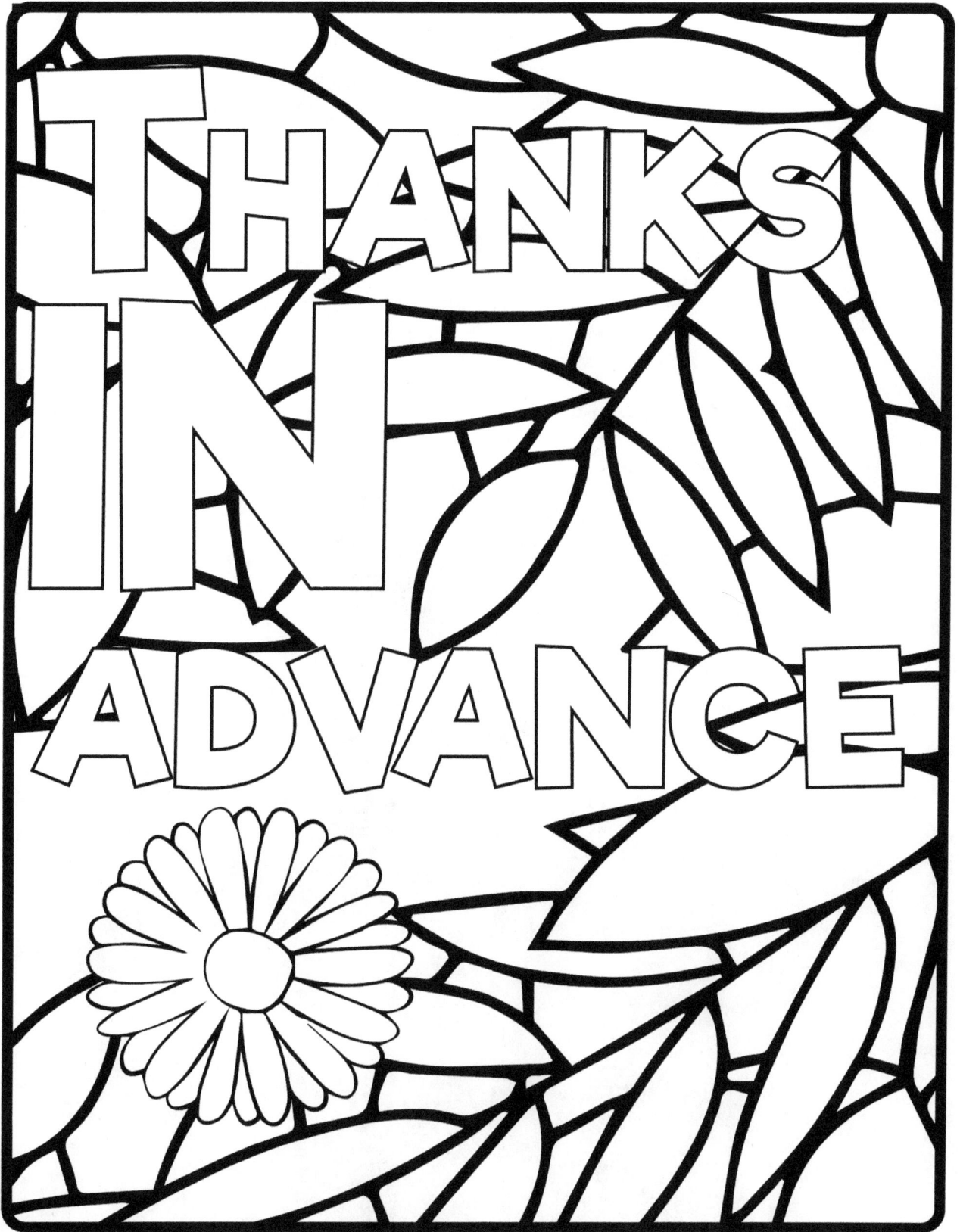

THANKS IN ADVANCE

♥ thank you for your purchase!

Tattoos can increase feelings of confidence and improve self-image. Some feel that their tattoos allow them to look more like who they feel on the inside. If you found any tattoo that you liked in this book, please consider sharing your artwork with us and others who may benefit from it.

Your support means the world to us!

leave a review ♥

www.ingramcontent.com/pod-product-compliance
Lightning Source LLC
Chambersburg PA
CBHW052116020426
42335CB00021B/2781